AF710375

International Research in Nutrition

Editor
BRITA ROLANDER-CHILÒ
Nutrition Foundation of Italy

PERGAMON PRESS
Oxford · New York · Toronto · Sydney · Paris · Frankfurt

U.K.	Pergamon Press Ltd., Headington Hill Hall, Oxford OX3 0BW, England
U.S.A.	Pergamon Press Inc., Maxwell House, Fairview Park, Elmsford, New York 10523, U.S.A.
CANADA	Pergamon of Canada, Suite 104, 150 Consumers Road, Willowdale, Ontario M2J 1P9, Canada
AUSTRALIA	Pergamon Press (Aust.) Pty. Ltd., P.O. Box 544, Potts Point, N.S.W. 2011, Australia
FRANCE	Pergamon Press SARL, 24 rue des Ecoles, 75240 Paris, Cedex 05, France
FEDERAL REPUBLIC OF GERMANY	Pergamon Press GmbH, 6242 Kronberg-Taunus, Pferdstrasse 1, Federal Republic of Germany

Copyright © 1979 Pergamon Press Ltd.

All Rights Reserved. No part of this publication may be reproduced, stored in a retrieval system or transmitted in any form or by any means: electronic, electrostatic, magnetic tape, mechanical, photocopying, recording or otherwise, without permission in writing from the publishers.

First edition 1979

TX
367
.I57
1979

British Library Cataloguing in Publication Data

International research in nutrition. -
(International research in nutrition and
food toxicology).
1. Nutrition - Research - Congresses
I. Rolander-Chilò, Brita
II. Nutrition Foundation of Italy
III. Series
641.1'07'2 TX367 79-40073
ISBN 0-08-024399-1

Printed in Great Britain by Biddles Ltd, Guildford, Surrey

Contents

Preface

The present volume includes the contributions to the First International Meeting organized by the Nutrition Foundation of Italy a few months after the official opening in 1977.

The young Italian Foundation has invited representations of similar organizations from the major countries in order to discuss the present status of nutritional research and teaching in the world and the priorities for future co-operative efforts.

The Group of Nutrition Foundations founded in Milan during this meeting is an original contribution to the field of nutrition and it may represent in the future a valuable support for the scientific communities in this critical area.

The present volume represents an effort to outline in a clear and comprehensive style the present status of the art and the most needed effort for the future.

In a rather concise form some of the leaders in nutrition research present for each country the results obtained, the different means used, the common or specific difficulties for any nutrition research and the distribution of scientific information among scientists, the medical professors and the public in this area of growing interest and still in need of experts, scientists and educators.

We are therefore particularly grateful to the contributors and to Mrs. Brita Rolander-Chilò, Secretary General of the Italian Foundation, who has organized the meeting and carefully edited the proceedings.

Milano, June 1978

PROFESSOR RODOLFO PAOLETTI
PRESIDENT
NUTRITION FOUNDATION OF ITALY

A New Organization: The Nutrition Foundation of Italy

Rodolfo Paoletti

Institute of Pharmacology and Pharmacognosy,
University of Milan, Italy
President, NFI

The Nutrition Foundation of Italy, the host of this Symposium, is the youngest among the world foundations because it has been charted on December 23, 1976.

I have therefore the challenging task not to discuss achievements — or failures — but to underline the proposed activities for the immediate and not so immediate future.

As Professor Alfredo Rabbi has mentioned in his introductory remarks to the present Symposium the Italian society faces two types of problems: insufficient alimentary resources for a still growing population of almost 60 million people and lack of interest and widespread knowledge — at least until very recently — for the complex scientific and technological problems involving food production, food safety and nutrition.

Our Foundation has been established to help the government, the academic and public organizations and the industry to solve these problems. Its focus will be therefore on science and education.

According to its chart to obtain its objectives the Foundation's functions are:

(a) to contribute to the education of medical doctors, biologists, pharmacists, investigators, paramedical personnel, teachers and the general public in the area of nutrition;

(b) to consult and interact with the government bodies and with the central and peripheral administrations with foreign government and with international and supernational organizations;

(c) to provide scientific information and support to the food industry in technological, toxicological and biomedical problems, in selected programmes of technological and health research, and in establishing better links on the international developments in the industrial production of food and in the science of nutrition;

(d) to publish specialized journals and reports and to prepare documents for the mass media and the public;

(e) to organize specialized meetings and courses for the scientists, technologists and executives of the food industry and industry in related areas and for the scientific community;

(f) to establish *ad hoc* committees for meetings, publications of journals, magazines and proceedings of scientific meetings and for the distribution of fellowships, grants and prizes.

The first activity planned by the Foundation has been—quite naturally—to organize the present symposium in order to evaluate the achievements of the different nutrition foundations in Europe and in America and to plan collaborative efforts for the future.

This Symposium will be followed in 1978 by an international meeting on "Chemical Toxicology of Food". This area of great concern in all the industrialized societies is of particular interest to Italy, a country which imports a considerable percentage of food raw material and which also exports a remarkable part of its food products.

Recent episodes involving industry, the government and the courts have underlined that the Italian laws are insufficient in this important area and should be updated possibly with the help of Italian and international experts.

The area of food toxicology research, information to the public, the government bodies, the scientific community will be covered in our proposed symposium.

This international meeting will be divided into different sections: safety assessment, legislation, toxicological evaluation of food additives, toxicology and nutrition and applied aspects of food toxicology.

Experts from many relevant disciplines have already been invited in each section and a truly international participation is assured. The proceedings will hopefully represent a useful contribution for specialists and administrators in the industrialized and raw-material-producing countries for several years. A symposium on the metabolic effects of ethanol is also planned for June 1979.

In addition to a yearly symposium on food toxicology and metabolism, special emphasis will be placed on the development of food toxicology in Italy.

Post-doctoral fellowships for specialization and research in toxicology are planned in order to encourage young scientists in Italy to enter this important field where the number of specialists is still insufficient in most countries.

In collaboration with the Toxicology section of the IUPHAR (International Union of Pharmacologists) and with the World Health Organization of Geneva, the NFI is also actively planning for the period 1978-1981 regular post-graduate courses on toxicology with an international staff and open to young scientists with chemical and biomedical background of Europe and the Americas and the emerging nations of Asia and Africa. The courses are also considered to be timely because of the introduction in the United States of the Toxicology Act which will considerably affect food imports and exports between the United States and other countries, including Italy.

The publication of textbooks, monographs and proceedings of meetings and courses is also an important part of the Foundation's activity.

The Italian edition of the well-known textbook produced by the American Nutrition Foundation, *Present Knowledges in Nutrition,* is in preparation, as well as the publication of two monographs on food additives and colorants prepared by Dr. Gaston Vettorazzi, the well-known expert of WHO in these areas.

A series of monographs for investigators and students and a newsletter are also in the planning stage.

Other activities will also be designed in collaboration with the other Nutrition Foundations in the frame of the newly established International Group, European—North American Section.

We are therefore confident that our new Foundation—in spite of the present difficulties in Italy—will represent a useful addition to the growing and active family of Nutrition Foundations of the World.

Introductory Remarks

William J. Darby

President, The Nutrition Foundation (USA)

Some of us have just arrived from a meeting in Sweden that marked the 500th anniversary year of the great University of Uppsala. We are, therefore, especially conscious of the fundamental roles of the university in society and of the gradual evolution of the university as an institution.

The modern university began to take form during the twelfth century and emerged from the church-related function of educating priests and monks beyond the level of monastic or cathedral schools. The concept of the university was a continuum of the formal institutionalized educational complex that may be traced to the earliest civilizations of Egypt, Mesopotamia and other cultures. The institutions that flowered during the Renaissance drew heavily upon the precedents for preservation and advancement of knowledge established by the ancient Greeks and Romans and by the Islamic universities.

The Foundation is a much newer instrument developed by society for the advancement of knowledge, education and the public good. Single-purpose support in perpetuity for charitable purposes, for relief, for a museum, for ecclesiastical interest, or for an academy of library began as early as the times of ancient Egypt, Greece and Rome. The modern version of the foundation, however, is predominantly a twentieth-century phenomenon.

> Today's American philanthropic foundation, with its profound impact upon society, dates from the gift of the English scientist, James Smithson, which resulted in the creation of the Smithsonian Institution in 1846. The influence of the foundation in the early twentieth century was characterized by the beneficial impact upon

research and education supported by large foundations with enormous resources. These foundations possessed broad purposes and flexibility of action assured by an automony of organization. These organized philanthropies, devoted to public good, were endowed with the fortunes of many who had attained great wealth in industry—notably, Andrew Carnegie, John D. Rockefeller, Jr., George Peabody, later Henry Ford, and numerous others. Their contributions to the public good represent one of the great benefits that result from our system of free enterprise. No other system has contributed so widely and wisely to the benefit of mankind.

In the preface to the recently published history of The Nutrition Foundation I quoted in part Dr. Allen Gregg, a distinguished Director of The Rockefeller Foundation, who wrote in 1941, the year that The Nutrition Foundation was chartered:

"If we take research in medicine to be the function we wish to preserve, we must be prepared to see new institutions appear for this purpose. Indeed, within the past forty years or less a new form of institution has appeared. The older institution is the university, the new institution is the foundation; the ground they have in common is the furtherance of medical research . . . .

"A foundation obviously may be more flexible and adaptable in its choice of research to be supported than is a university which is responsible for maintaining established teaching personnel and for preserving knowledge as well as discovering it . . . .

"Compared with a government's subsidizing of research, foundations can much more easily work outside national boundaries and support demonstrations of theories not widely enough accepted or fully enough proven to qualify for government support . . . they are rarely able to expand on the scale now characteristic of government . . . .

"Compared with learned societies foundations have a much wider choice of fields to aid and are less dominated by specialist or partisan interests . . . .

"In contrast to the individual private donor the foundation is more deliberate, sustained, and dependable, better advised and less personal . . . .

> "Foundations vary with their age, their size, the current economic conditions, their form of organization, their general purposes and their specific fields of interest . . . with the personal qualifications and characters of their officers and trustees . . . .
>
> "The first ten years of a foundation's existence determine in large manner its general policies over a much longer period of time. Though resolutely struggling against the formation of tradition the first officers develop precedents and usages in spite of themselves . . . and the first ten years are delightful in the opportunity they afford . . . ."

It is this opportunity that makes the occasion of establishing the Nutrition Foundation of Italy such an exciting and promising event. As we anticipate these opportunities and responsibilities it is well for us to be mindful of the heritage of the Foundation concept, its decided influences on research and education—contributions to the public good that represent one of the great benefits of a system of free enterprise.

Apparent on every hand, nationally and internationally, are beneficial influences of these philanthropic foundations. These influences are felt in scientific development; medical knowledge and health care; the humanities, arts and human relations; agriculture and food production; education; and the upgrading of the general quality of life.

The programs of the major foundations have been supported by enormous resources endowed from personal fortunes of individuals who amassed their fortunes in industry. The growth and maturity of industry within the capitalistic system is marked by its increasing social awareness, and the development of a high sense of corporate citizenship by leading industrial executives.

The Nutrition Foundation concept is a superb example of the recognized social responsibility of the food and allied industries and of the willingness of highly responsible corporations and executives to accept this responsibility by corporate support of research, education and public service in science, medicine, public health and social welfare, free from any self-serving motivation.

I congratulate the industrial and scientific leaders in Italy for their public-spirited action in founding this latest in the growing group of national Nutrition Foundations, and thus providing an expansion of the opportunities for enhanced communication and exchange among existing Nutrition Foundations in order that we all may contribute maximally to furthering the health of mankind through increased basic and applied knowledge of nutrition and foods.

Thank you for the privilege of participating in this meeting.

Reference

King, Charles Glen, *A Good Idea: The History of the Nutrition Foundation,* The Nutrition Foundation, New York and Washington, 1976.

Introductory Remarks

Alfredo Rabbi

President, The National Institute of Nutrition, Rome, Italy

It is with great pleasure that I have accepted the invitation of Professor Paoletti to participate at this Meeting of "The Nutrition Foundations and the International Research in Nutrition".

As President of the National Institute of Nutrition, an organism of the Italian government depending in particular on the Ministry of Agriculture, I greatly appreciate this opportunity, and I wish to address my personal welcome to the distinguished investigators here convened.

Italy, as we all know, owns an important tradition of nutritional studies. Recently, in the issue of December 1976, the *Nutrition Reviews* reported a chronology of events in the development and application in the science of nutrition. Such report mentions some Italian investigators in the nutritional research: among those, Sanctorius, who published the first metabolic balance study; Bartolotti, the discoverer of milk sugar; Menghini, who found that the iron content of blood could be increased by feeding iron-rich-containing foods; Frapolli, who described and named pellagra and Marzari who believed maize the cause of that disease.

But let me go on a little more with this Italian spirit and here remember Spallanzani, Beccari, Albertoni, Luciani, Baglioni, Visco, Quagliarello, Bergami . . . .

The science of nutrition in Italy is still the subject of important studies. Even if our Italian universities have been reluctant to establish chairs and institutes of Nutrition, nevertheless this science is being taught. Much less care, unfortunately, is given to the teaching of nutrition in elementary and secondary schools, where it should receive particular emphasis.

Such a low general level of nutritional information is a severe limit to our fellow-citizens; this limit is also present in high-cultured people since, as it is well known, culture in Italy is mainly oriented in a humanistic and artistic direction: Italy is a country in which the "two cultures" are not present.

The consequence of this situation is the permanence of prejudices and habits, most of the time wrong, complicating the alimentary problems of our country. As you know, in Italy the economic difficulties depend on a transformation economy, on the absence of raw materials and an unfavourable ratio of population to agricultural surface; every Italian has a share of 0.3 hectar of soil, of which only 800 square meters are of high productivity.

The task of the Italian nutritionist is therefore very difficult in this time of economic crisis, particularly from the point of view of information and divulgation.

This is the reason why we welcome and encourage any enterprise in our country, such as this one, that might bring to a better perspective the nutritional problems.

Philosophy and Program of the Nutrition Foundation

William J. Darby

The Nutrition Foundation (USA)

Background and Organization

The concept central to the organization of The Nutrition Foundation was expressed by Mr. Clarence Francis, former President of General Foods Corporation, community leader of renown, and one of the two initiators of the Foundation. He recalled that in 1938 ". . . we were searching for an activity on which the industry should and would act in the public welfare". This action took concrete form in December 1941 with the chartering of The Nutrition Foundation. The initial Board of Trustees consisted of top-level executives of fifteen major food and food-related companies with a sincere motivation of public service.

To forestall an anticipated public doubt that ". . . profit-minded industry would be unselfish enough to spend time and money on anything that detracted from profits . . ." they procured as their Chairman a man from outside of industry whose character and reputation were beyond reproach; they developed an organization with bylaws and controls that would assure that monies contributed by industry would be used to the benefit of the public, and sought to support the independent work of the most capable research personnel anywhere in the world. A distinguished non-industrial, academic scientist, Dr. Charles Glen King, was chosen as Scientific Director (later, President) of the Foundation and twelve Public Members were elected to the Board of Trustees. These exceptional men were presidents of major educational institutions or of Foundations, responsible government officials in health (the Surgeon General of the United States) or agriculture (Chief, Nutrition Section, U.S. Department of agriculture), or religious leaders. The number and role of Public Members was subsequently expanded. In 1971 bylaw and organization changes made Public Members the majority on the Executive Committee of the Trustees and Chairmen of the Board and of the Executive Committee.

At its first meeting the Trustees approved the recommendation of the new Director, Dr. C. G. King, for a general program of scientific action by the Foundation:

> "(1) Scientific research, on a long-range basis, to discover new fundamental knowledge in the field embraced by the science of nutrition, for better public health; (2) scientific research on a current basis, to solve immediate public health problems in that field; (3) scientific research on a war basis to aid our government in dealing with emergency problems in that field, for education purposes, in order that the science of nutrition may be more effectively applied for better public health."

Dr. King's recommendations reflected the purposes set forth in the charter of The Nutrition Foundation:

> (1) to develop and apply the science of nutrition, in its fundamental conception and practical significance as a basic science of public health;
>
> (2) to aid the food industry in appropriately solving its general and individual problems relating to that science; and
>
> (3) to do so by lawful and effective means, as a public institution operated on a non-profit basis and dedicated to improve the food and diet and thus to better the health of the people of the United States of America.

Early Grant Program

The Foundation's initial research grant program, reviewed and recommended by fifteen of the best US and Canadian scientists who served as the Scientific Advisory Committee, supported research in human requirements for specific nutrients, functions of individual nutrients, maternal and infant nutrition, direct public health problems, educational and professional training and war-time nutrition needs.

Foundation funds supported pioneer studies of human requirements of essential amino acids by W. C. Rose; investigations on methionine, choline and labile methyl metabolism by Vincent du Vigneaud; nutritional genetics research by George Beadle and E. L. Tatum; a cooperative comparison of the composition and nutritional values of human and of cow's milk by L. A. Maynard, Icie Macy Hoobler and H. L. Longenecker; nutritive value studies on hardened (hydrogenated) fats; nutritive values of military rations; comparative studies of the nutrient composition of various processed foods and the effects of processing technics on nutritive values; metabolic and nutritional importance of stress (including starvation); nutritional factors in dental caries. I may note that seven scientists who early in their careers received crucial grant support from The Nutrition Foundation subsequently have been selected as Nobel Laureates.

To provide national nutrition advisory leadership the Foundation, at the request of the National Academy of Sciences, joined with two other foundations in supporting the establishment of the Food and Nutrition Board of the National Academy of Sciences-National Research Council. The national and international contributions of this Board and of its constituent committees, especially the Food Protection Committee and its Food Chemical Codex, and the Committee on Dietary Allowances, serve as examples of the effective catalytic roles that a small, specialized foundation can serve through providing modest enabling grants to initiate a needed organization or development. The Nutrition Foundation has played a similar catalytic role in the organization and program development of the International Union of Nutritional Sciences (IUNS), the Protein Advisory Group (PAG), the Society for Nutrition Education and its *Journal of Nutrition Education,* and the National Nutrition Consortium.

The wide spectrum of research supported by The Nutrition Foundation is well summarized and documented in the History of the Foundation with its listing of 550 publications as examples. Among these are key studies on newly identified essential nutrients, the relationship between nutrition and intellectual development, chemical senses (taste and smell), appetite, nutrition and cancer, nutritional toxicology, trace elements, fiber, and biological availability, to mention but a few. The total grant support of some $17 million is small but has proved important in stimulating the opening of many new interests that subsequently have received major funding from other, usually governmental, sources.

Nutrition Reviews

When The Nutrition Foundation was organized research findings were being published in widely diverse journals often without competent, critical, nutritionally knowledgeable editorial reviews. *The Journal of Nutrition* was the only US journal in the field at that time and the *British Journal of Nutrition* was not founded until 1947. A publication was needed that would critically and continuously review current research reports relating to nutrition, including brief authoritative critical reviews which placed current research in perspective as to its importance, validity and application. With approval of the Scientific Advisory Committee, The Nutrition Foundation accepted the challenge to support such a monthly journal, set up an independent editorial office and board of academic scientists, and initiated publication of the new journal, *Nutrition Reviews,* in November 1942.

The journal maintains a world-wide circulation and is recognized today as an outstanding contribution to professional and lay education as well as research. Subscriptions to the journal provide only about one-half the cost; the balance is subsidized by The Nutrition Foundation. The journal carries no commercial advertising.

An important outgrowth of *Nutrition Reviews* has been the book *Present Knowledge in Nutrition*—a series of succinct, authoritative documented chapters on basic and applied nutrition. This work serves as a standard supplementary text for many upper-level and graduate courses in nutrition as well as a reference work for scholars and teachers at several levels. It also offers media communicators authoritative background on specific subjects and issues. More than 10,000 copies of the third edition were distributed. The new fourth edition, published some 8 months ago, has already had sales of well over 5000, is stocked in many university bookstores, and is being translated into Spanish (by INCAP) and Portuguese. Dr. Paoletti has received permission for the new Nutrition Foundation of Italy to translate it into Italian, and negotiations are underway for a French translation.

Special numbers or Supplements of *Nutrition Reviews* are published occasionally to consolidate current information relating to a rapidly developing topic, to make accessible material otherwise difficult to obtain, or to provide needed objective scientific assessment of controversial claims widely disseminated to the public. An example of the latter is the special supplement published in 1974 on food faddism and nutrition misinformation, over 70,000 copies of which have been distributed. A more recent example is the publication and distribution of the Marabou Conference report on the role of fiber in nutrition in co-operation with the Swedish and British Nutrition Foundations.

Symposia and Monographs

Through its symposium and monograph series, the Foundation is establishing benchmarks for research development in newly explored scientific areas of nutrition especially applicable to human health and disease. A series of international conferences arranged within universities are supported by The Nutrition Foundation. These conferences deal broadly with selected subject areas of wide interest; review the existing knowledge of the particular subject; identify areas in which research is needed; and indicate ways in which the knowledge gained from research can be applied to benefit man. The critically edited papers of each symposium are published as a monograph, three of which are now available:

Sugars in Nutrition,

Protein-Calorie Malnutrition,

Trace Elements in Human Health and Disease (Vols. 1 and 2).

Two additional monographs will be published in 1977:

Chemical Senses in Nutrition, edited by Dr. Morley Kare,

Nutrition and Drug Interrelations, edited by Dr. Julius M. Coon and Dr. John Hathcock.

Symposia on these latter two subjects were held in 1976. The manuscripts of an international conference on Fermented Food Beverages in Nutrition held June 15-17, 1977 at Rochester, Minnesota, are now being edited for publication. A symposium on infant feeding is under development and is scheduled late in 1978 at Michigan State University.

The gratifyingly large demand for published monographs and the laudatory reviews provide evidence of the quality and value of this program. The monographs are effectively used by those who plan the translation of science through forums and for popular scientific and medical informational programs.

The Foundation staff also cooperates in the planning and staging of similar, but less broad conferences supported primarily by other institutions. The Foundation recently has cooperated in the planning of two international conferences, one on fiber and another on obesity, supported by and hosted at the National Institutes of Health. The meeting on fiber has been held, the congress on obesity will take place in Washington, DC, October 20-26, 1977. Proceedings of both conferences will be published. Through cooperative efforts with other nutrition foundations, the NIH, scientific, professional and medical societies, the National Academy of Sciences, international organizations, industry and its associations and governmental and legislative bodies, The Nutrition Foundation serves continuously as a major national scientific resource specializing in basic and applied food science and human nutrition.

Personnel Development and Recognition Awards

Emphasis on identifying and facilitating the growth of especially promising young nutrition scientists has characterized the grant program of The Nutrition Foundation. The Future Leaders Awards are designed for this purpose. These grants of up to $10,000 annually for 2 to 3 years support the research of young doctorate-level scientists holding their first academic appointments. Among the seventy-eight recipients since 1964 are Myron Winick, Quinton Rogers, Barbara Underwood, Harold Sandstead, Oscar Pineda, Charles Halsted, Johanna Dwyer, to identify but a few.

To identify nutrition as a subspeciality in medicine and encourage development of personnel in the medical area, The Nutrition Foundation provides grant funds to the American College of Physicians annually to select and award 2-, 3-year scholarships to selected, competent young internists with special interest in nutrition. Many years ago the Foundation, in cooperation with the American Medical Association, supported the initial Goldberger Fellowships for medical students interested in nutrition. This activity has now been expanded and is completely funded by the AMA.

Since 1948-1949 the Foundation has supported four annual awards to recognize outstanding contributors to nutrition knowledge through research. They are the Osborne and Mendel Award of the American Institute of Nutrition; the Babcock-Hart Award of the Institute of Food Technologists; the Mary Swartz Rose Award of the American Dietetic Association; and the Goldberger Award in Clinical Nutrition of the American Medical Association. The latter association has recently assumed the financial responsibility for the Goldberger Award. The Foundation has just announced the establishment of the William C. Rose Lectureship in Biochemistry and Nutrition, an annual national lectureship to recognize those qualities of scientific and personal leadership of Professor Rose.

Such Foundation activities are important forces in setting the quality of scholarship in nutrition sciences.

Nutrition Education in Medicine

Just 5 years ago we joined with other agencies in sponsoring a second national conference on nutrition education in medical schools. At that time faculty members from but six of the nation's medical schools spoke of active teaching programs in their institutions. In reviewing the financing of nutrition education I noted that although the NIH long has provided important support for research, it had not provided funds for the training of medical students in nutrition. Since that time we have tirelessly pressed for making federal support available for this purpose.

Five of the six programs then existing (1972—Vanderbilt University, University of Alabama, Tulane, Mt. Sinai, Columbia University and University of Missouri) had been significantly supported or initiated by grants from The Nutrition Foundation.

The resultant widespread interest in this subject was evidenced immediately by a great demand for the published proceedings of the conference; over 4000 copies have been distributed upon request. More significantly, we have received numerous thoughtfully prepared requests for financial support, advice and consultation in establishing programs.

The Nutrition Foundation has since responded by awarding six critically selected educational grants-in-aid to establish programs in medical centers, and by stimulating funding for programs from other sources and catalyzing communication between and among medical schools. The most recent grant, a 5-year $1 million one to the University of Pittsburgh, was made possible by a generous gift to The Nutrition Foundation from the Howard Heinz Endowment. The Foundation staff has been directly involved in planning, counseling and implementing important developments financed by other foundations that in turn often were directly stimulated by our successful involvement in the field. Simultaneously, members of The Nutrition Foundation's staff have participated in regional and university-based seminars, symposia, advisory committee sessions, clinics, lectureships and even courses in at least half of the nation's medical schools.

The placement of Future Leaders Awards for young faculty members and of the Scholars in medical nutrition selected by the prestigious American College of Physicians strengthens efforts to integrate nutrition teaching in the medical curriculum.

In recognition of the need for modern, authoritative, effective teaching materials for use in this overall development, The Nutrition Foundation has produced a series of resources:

A new clinical section in *Nutrition Reviews.*

The new edition of *Nutrition Reviews'* "Present Knowledge in Nutrition".

A series of teaching aids—slides, special pamphlets, audiotapes, prototype lectures—under continuing development by the Foundation in collaboration with and support from a variety of organizations and institutions—including Helen Keller International, USAID, UNICEF, and commercial producers and distributors of educational materials for post-graduate or continuing education.

A detailed curriculum for nutrition in a community health teaching program designed by Dr. Reva Frankle.

An annotated bibliography of nutrition education in medical schools, prepared and published under contract with Health Manpower of HEW.

A selected bibliography of source materials for physicians and students.

What is the effectiveness of these efforts? A recent survey by our staff of offerings and developments in medical schools in the United States identified twenty-nine schools as having significant *required* instruction in nutrition. The Nutrition Foundation has been an important influence through direct support to or advisory involvement with this development in nineteen of the twenty-nine schools. Seventy-three of eighty schools surveyed indicate that they now have elective courses in nutrition for medical students. This is obviously rewarding progress.

The task is *not* complete, however; the depth and scope of many of the electives do not afford desirably comprehensive background. Primarily only those schools assisted by The Nutrition Foundation have established meaningful clinical laboratory services to assess nutriture. We hope that the recent grant to the University of Pittsburgh will result in establishing a major pacesetting, well-balanced center in nutrition offering senior leaderships in clinical, biochemical, dietary and applied nutrition, and a versatile, well-organized nutrition laboratory for patient diagnosis and monitoring. Such a major center should have great effectiveness in postgraduate or continuing education of the physician as well as in undergraduate training. Its presence will challenge and stimulate other medical centers to raise their standards of nutrition education and service.

Public Issues

The Nutrition Foundation undertakes objective analysis and assessment of the scientific evidence concerning selected public issues. Its organization, research experience and resources make it an especially effective vehicle for developing coordinated research studies critically designed and executed by academic scientists with impeccable qualifications. There is long precedent for The Nutrition Foundation serving this role through the utilization of special grant funds to further knowledge and understanding of research interests relating to issues of public concern. A current example may be cited: when the untested hypothesis of Dr. Benjamin Feingold concerning the possibility that certain foods and/or food additives might be factors in the syndrome of hyperkinesis was popularized, the Foundation undertook the task of obtaining an authoritative assessment of the available factual information and sought expert guidance as to desirable program activities which might usefully be undertaken to clarify the issue.

Toward this end, the Foundation established the National Advisory Committee on Hyperkinesis, the first report of which was published June 1975. Immediately thereafter two other committees were activated—one, a committee of the Board of Trustees with responsibility for obtaining special funding to support a coordinated research program as recommended by the National Advisory Committee; the other, a committee of food scientists, primarily industry-based, to develop appropriate challenge and placebo foodstuffs to be utilized in double blind studies to test the Feingold hypothesis. This latter committee skillfully developed and tested identical, acceptable test foodstuffs as recommended by the National Advisory Committee and supervised the preparation and planned distribution of these challenge foods to selected, approved investigators whose protocols have been approved by the National Advisory Committee.

The Nutrition Foundation has received applications for a supply of challenge foods and for grant support from investigators from a variety of centers in the US and Canada. All requests approved to date by the National Advisory Committee have been funded and research progress has been such that an interim report was released in June, 1977. A full committee review and report should be made early in 1978.

We currently are organizing a similar review of US Dietary Goals.

Restatement of Objectives and Functions

During the past year a panel of our Trustees has, at my request, examined all aspects of The Nutrition Foundation's program. They have carefully restated and clarified the objectives and functions as follows:

The Nutrition Foundation's basic objective is the advancement of the knowledge of food and nutrition and its effective application in improving health and welfare. To attain this objective, the Nutrition Foundation's functions are:

> to identify, define and selectively promote the support of needed research in the field of nutrition and the nutritional value of food, as well as food safety and acceptability as influenced by current and developing technology;
>
> to assist in the development of personnel, libraries and media of scientific communication in order to advance research and the application of knowledge in nutrition;
>
> to promote the exchange, coordination and assessment of scientific information through continuous communications with other agencies and institutions by means of symposia and workshops that explore critical problems and existing knowledge in nutrition, nationally and internationally;
>
> to encourage and effect the adoption of adequate nutrition curricula in medical schools and throughout the formal education system;
>
> to disseminate nutrition knowledge through the most appropriate channels of communication, both professional and public;
>
> to serve as a public resource for identifying, collating and obtaining authoritative assessment and interpretation of scientific information on issues pertaining to nutritional values and food safety.
>
> The panel recommended that, in the future:
>
> The Foundation should conduct more active public information campaigns on relevant issues, including such activities as the holding of public forums and seminars, holding press conferences on occasion, the issuing of releases, liaison with media involving preparation of major articles, the appearance on television and radio shows and the taking of public policy positions.
>
> Additional, occasional summary reports, of a news rather than technical nature, should be prepared and sent to friends of the

Foundation in academia, government, and the public sector who should be interested in and kept informed of the Foundation's activities. These would be in addition to present activities in the field of publications.

The panel requested that a study be made of advisability of a preponderance of Future Leader support, with emphasis on research in the broad field of the nutritional effects of food processing, distribution and preparation. Considerations of food safety, additives, naturally occurring non-nutrients, risk-benefit and other matters relating to the availability and acceptability of foods should be studied. This study is underway.

I hope that this incomplete overview of The Nutrition Foundation's activities, the changes in emphasis in response to public needs and available resources, and our outlook for the future may be useful to you. I look forward to the reviews of other programs here and in the future to bring all of us nearer our goal of "advancement of knowledge of food and nutrition and its effective application in improving the health and welfare of mankind".

Reference

King, Charles Glen, *A Good Idea: The History of the Nutrition Foundation,* The Nutrition Foundation, New York and Washington, 1976.

An International Group of National Nutrition Foundations European—North American Section

William J. Darby

President, The Nutrition Foundation (USA)

The number of national nutrition foundations with similar objectives and functions is increasing. Their broad common objective is to advance the knowledge of food and nutrition and its effective application in improving the health and welfare of mankind. While programs of individual foundations vary according to their size and established priorities, all are concerned with promotion of research, with general and professional education, and may serve public advisory roles by drawing on knowledgeable sources of scientific information in government, industry and the academic community.

Involvement of responsible academic scientists and public leaders in determining foundation policy assures independency of action and scientific objectivity free of any self interest of supporters. Each of the foundations serves the public as a non-profit institution. Their broad bases of support are derived in large measure, but not exclusively, from a variety of forward-looking food and food-related industries and other sources such as foundations, national governments, other public institutions and individual donors.

In recognition of these common features and the potential benefits from collaborative efforts toward attaining their broad objectives, The British Nutrition Foundation, The Swedish Nutrition Foundation and The Nutrition Foundation (USA) established during the Ninth International Congress of Nutrition in 1972 an informal collaboration to effect continuing communication regarding activities and events supported by the respective foundations, to exchange experiences, and to assist in the planning of certain future activities. The foundations have since exchanged formal reports and publications, calendars of scheduled events, and informal correspondence concerning future activities and other matters of mutual interest.

The foundations also have jointly planned and sponsored activities considered to be of international significance. Examples of jointly sponsored activities include:

The Nutrition Foundations' Reprints of exceptionally valuable classic books in the field of nutrition. The first in this series was Graham Lusk's *The Elements of the Science of Nutrition;* the second is Rosen Von Rosenstein's *Diseases of Children and their Remedies* (published to coincide with the 500th anniversary year of the University of Uppsala, Von Rosenstein's University).

The Nutrition Foundations' Book Award, established to recognize authoritative, exceptionally meritorious books dealing with major concepts of food and nutrition of interest to the non-specialist. The first title selected to receive this award was W. R. Aykroyd's *The Conquest of Famine* (English edition published by Chatto and Windus, London, 1974; American edition published by Readers Digest Press, New York, 1975). The second work selected is *Food: The Gift of Osiris* by William J. Darby, Paul Ghalioungui, and Louis Grivetti, Academic Press, London and New York. The Netherlands and Swiss Nutrition Foundations joined the Swedish and British Foundations in making the selection; all five of these Foundations are participating in the 1977 award.

Joint distribution through their respective subscription publications (BNF *Nutrition Bulletin,* Näringsforskning, *Nutrition Reviews*) of papers from a symposium in Stockholm concerning Fiber in Nutrition.

Preparation of a series of considered guidelines proposed to assure appropriate recognition of nutritional principles in the manufacturing of certain types of foods, "Proposed Nutritional Guidelines for Utilization of Industrially Produced Nutrients", William J. Darby and Leif Hambraeus, *Näringsforskning,* Arg. 19, 113-120, 1975.

Cooperative promotion of publications of the several foundations.

Mutual counsel in planning and selection of participants for symposia and obtaining needed materials, information or assessments of developments or personnel.

Encouragement and assistance in the development of new national nutrition foundations.

The reproduction or translation of scientific matter from one foundation source for publication by other foundations in their periodicals. Every effort is made to preserve the original meaning of articles and to credit the source.

Attendance of representatives of the collaborating foundations at meetings of the respective organizations has been encouraged in a manner not financially burdensome to the host foundations. Opportunities for joint meetings have thereby occurred at least annually.

This collaboration proved valuable to the three foundations initially involved. Their invitation for participation by other independent, public-oriented nutrition foundations has resulted in expansion of membership to include The Netherlands Nutrition Foundation, The Swiss Nutrition Foundation and The Nutrition Foundation of Italy.

In discussions at the Fourteenth Symposium of The Swedish Nutrition Foundation in Uppsala, June 20-22, 1977 and the initial Advisory Committee meeting of The Nutrition Foundation of Italy in Milan, June 27-28, 1977, representatives of the British, Netherlands, Italian, Swedish, Swiss and US Foundations agreed to continue this useful level of cooperation.

The planning of new selections for the Nutrition Foundations' Reprint Series and for The Nutrition Foundations' Book Award is underway; a forthcoming publication from The Nutrition Foundation of Italy will include summaries of the background organization and activities of the cooperating foundations; a broader exchange of national reports on scientific developments and issues, and Foundation publications and information was agreed upon; The Nutrition Foundation of

Italy announced plans to translate and publish the fourth edition of Nutrition Reviews' *Present Knowledge in Nutrition;* consideration was given to additional collaborative efforts. The possibility of a jointly sponsored international symposium to develop broad guidelines for assessing risk-benefit considerations relating to food safety, wholesomeness, nutritive values, availability, acceptability and needs is being considered. Differing needs of developing and of highly industrialized regions, urbanized and rural areas, and the cultural traditions and desires of individual societies would be recognized in any such discussions.

Finally, the representatives considered the most effective composition and size of the group in view of present resources, personnel and programs. They agreed that desirable expansion initially could most productively be on a regional basis, as demonstrated by the useful growth of the European—North American section, and suggested that other similar informal groups might profitably be developed in other regions (e.g. Western Hemispheric, Asian, etc.), as the Nutrition Foundation movement spreads. The individual member foundations expressed their eagerness to assist in developing new national Nutrition Foundations and effective liaison groups.

The British Nutrition Foundation

Sir David Cuthbertson

President of the Foundation

Introduction

It was during the early and middle sixties that the idea of establishing a British Nutrition Foundation was first suggested. A small group of industrialists, scientists and medical men held a series of meetings as a result of which the requirement for such a Foundation firmly emerged. They were conscious that during the Second World War a food and nutrition policy, which it can honestly be claimed was second to none in terms of its success, had been established and operated in the United Kingdom and it undoubtedly played a major part in the war effort.

However, quite rapidly after the war, when rationing ended, interest in nutrition as such tended to wane, partly because of the success of the wartime nutrition policy and the resultant improvements in the health, particularly of British children. It was thought, wrongly as it has subsequently been found, that all pressing problems of human nutrition had been solved. We had not understood that with freedom of food choice and affluence, different nutritional problems arise.

Consequently, there was a considerable period during which the importance of research, and particularly information and education in nutritional matters, took second or even lower place to other developments. The group of people to whom I have referred were conscious of this and determined to do something about it. I will not enumerate all the people in the group who did so much to get things moving but I should, I think, at least mention the late Sir Charles Dodds, and Mr. Joseph Rank, of Ranks Hovis McDougall, both of whom found the time in their busy lives to take a leading part in establishing the Foundation.

The group knew that the Nutrition Foundation Inc. had existed in the USA since 1941 and so early during their deliberations they invited Dr. Glen King, who had been a moving force in the Nutrition Foundation Inc., to attend one of their meetings in London. Very useful discussions took place and, while it was recognized that some aspects of the Nutrition Foundation Inc., would not particularly suit the specific requirements as seen in the United Kingdom, a great fund of information was gleaned and this was carefully sifted so as to arrive at the best answer which would suit the British scene.

And so it was that finally on February 15, 1967 the British Nutrition Foundation was formally established by the following nine Founder Member Companies:

Allied Farm Foods Limited
Beecham Group Limited
H. J. Heinz Company Limited
Marks & Spencer Limited
Ranks Hovis McDougall Limited
Schweppes (Home) Limited
Spillers Limited
Tate & Lyle Limited
Unilever Limited

Membership grew very rapidly and within a few years there were no less than fifty Member Companies. Over the years some of the smaller companies who were Members were taken over by larger companies and we have now stabilized at a membership of some 44 companies (see Table 1). However, we are hoping to increase on this during the next year or so and I will have more to say on that later.

Before telling you something of the objects of the BNF I must make reference to Professor Alastair Frazer who was closely involved in the initial setting up of the BNF. The Foundation was very fortunate in securing him as its first Director-General. As you know he was a brilliant medical scientist of international repute. However, in addition to that, and fortunately for us, he had many contacts in the food industry and a considerable knowledge of its problems and how it operates. Under his dynamic leadership the Foundation got off to an excellent start but, most regrettably, he died suddenly in June 1969. He was sadly missed

Table 1

Member Companies *(as at 1st September 1977)*

Associated British Foods Limited	*Kraft Foods Limited*
Beecham Group Limited	*J. Lyons & Company Limited*
BP Proteins Limited	*Marks & Spencer Limited*
British Arkady Company Limited (The)	*Mars Limited*
British Home Stores Limited	*Metal Box Limited*
British Soya Products Limited	*Milk Marketing Board (The)*
British Sugar Corporation Limited	*Nabisco Limited*
Brooke Bond Liebig Services Limited	*Nestle Company Limited (The)*
Cadbury Schweppes Limited	*Potato Marketing Board*
Coca-Cola Export Corporation (The)	*Ranks Hovis McDougall Limited*
COOP Denmark	*Reckitt & Colman Limited*
CPC (United Kingdom) Limited	*Robertson Foods Limited*
Distillers Company (Yeast) Limited (The)	*Roche Products Limited*
FMC Limited	*J. Sainsbury Limited*
Fresh Fruit & Vegetable Information Bureau (The)	*Scottish Milk Marketing Board (The)*
	Slimming Magazine Limited
H. J. Heinz Company Limited	*Spillers Limited*
Imperial Chemical Industries Limited	*Tate & Lyle Limited*
Imperial Foods Limited	*Unigate Limited*
Kellogg Company of Great Britain, Limited	*Unilever Limited*
	Union International Company Limited (The)
	United Biscuits (Holdings) Limited
	Weetabix Limited
	Whitbread & Company Limited
	Whitworths Holdings Limited

and it took some time before the Foundation regained the impetus which he had imparted to it.

Objects of the British Nutrition Foundation

Against this background, I would now like to quote for you the objects for which the Foundation was established as stated in our Memorandum and Articles of Association. These, you will appreciate, are in legal parlance and I trust you will bear with me. They are:

(A) To carry out, and to advance, promote or procure the carrying out of, scientific research and investigation into the values of edible and potable substances of every description as food and the effect thereof on the consumer and the utilization of ingredients in, and methods of and processes for cultivating, manufacturing, producing, preparing, preserving, packaging or marketing or distributing (whether wholesale or retail), such substances with a view to the preservation or improvement of the health of the consumer, and to make available to the public the results of such scientific research and investigation by all methods which may seem appropriate including (but without prejudice to the generality of the foregoing) by means of meetings, conferences, oral communications, written publications, advertisements and sound and television broadcasting.

(B) To undertake, and to advance, promote or procure, the training and education of any persons with a view to their being able to carry out, or to train or educate others to carry out, such scientific research and investigation as is referred to in sub-paragraph (A) above.

(C) To undertake, and to advance, promote or procure, by all available means the education of the public in nutrition and the dissemination of information relating to nutrition.

In simple terms, and laymen's language, these can be briefly summarized as follows:

(A) to promote research in nutrition,
(B) to disseminate information in nutritional matters,
(C) to encourage education in nutritional matters.

These then are the three main areas in which the British Nutrition Foundation operates—Research, Information and Education—and I would like to outline for you, briefly, our activities in these spheres.

However, before doing so, I think I should first explain how the Foundation is organized and how it uses its committee structure.

Organization of the BNF

The Officers

The Officers are:

(a) *The President*

This is the position that at present I have the honour of holding. My predecessor for the period 1970-1976 was Professor Sir Frank

Young who is well known to many of you. He was appointed the first President early in 1970, some time after Professor Alastair Frazer, the first Director-General, had died, and at about the same time as Miss Dorothy Hollingsworth was appointed as Director-General.

(b) *The Chairman*

(i) The Chairman is elected annually for a period of 1 year though there is provision in the Articles of Association whereby he may serve for a maximum period of 2 years.

(ii) The appointment rotates between an Industrialist and a Scientist which has the very beneficial effect of ensuring that direction of the Foundation's affairs is well balanced and there is an absence of a permanent bias in policy matters.

(iii) The present Chairman is Professor J. C. Waterlow, CMG, who, as most of you know, is the Professor of Human Nutrition at the London School of Hygiene and Tropical Medicine.

(c) *The Vice-Chairman*

(i) As with the Chairman, this post rotates between an Industrialist and a Scientist so that if a Scientist is Chairman an Industrialist is Vice-Chairman and vice versa.

(ii) The present incumbent is Mr. Gordon L. Shemilt, DFC, a Director of Tate & Lyle Limited, and he will be taking over as Chairman from Professor J. C. Waterlow, CMG, at our Annual General Meeting on November 24, 1977.

(d) *The Honorary Treasurer*

The Honorary Treasurer is also elected annually and for the past 5 years this post has been held by Mr. Joseph Rank who is Chairman of Ranks Hovis McDougall Limited.

The above Officers are all part-time and unpaid. There are three Permanent Officers in the full-time employment of the Foundation and they are:

(a) Director-General: Miss Dorothy Hollingsworth, OBE

(b) Secretary to the Foundation and Membership Secretary: Mr. P. M. Victory, OBE, MC

(c) Senior Scientific Officer: Miss Elisabeth Morse

In support of them there is a small secretarial staff of four. Consequently, as you can see, we are a reasonably streamlined organization.

The Permanent Officers are kept very busy, particularly in work in Information and Education, and in servicing the Council and its Committees. A list of Officers and the Chairmen of Committees is at Table 2.

Table 2

Officers and Chairmen of Committees
(as at 1st September 1977)

Officers	
President	Sir David Cuthbertson, CBE, DSc, MD, FRCPE, FRSE (Honorary Senior Research Fellow in Pathological Biochemistry, University of Glasgow. Formerly Director of Rowett Research Institute)
Chairman of the Council	Professor J. C. Waterlow, CMG, MD, ScD, FRCP (Professor of Human Nutrition, London School of Hygiene & Tropical Medicine)
Vice-Chairman and Chairman Designate of the Council	Gordon L. Shemilt, DFC (Director, Tate & Lyle Limited)
Hon. Treasurer	Joseph Rank (Chairman, Ranks Hovis McDougall Limited)
Director-General	Miss Dorothy Hollingsworth, OBE, BSc, FRIC, FIBiol, FIFST, SRD
Secretary and Membership Secretary	P. M. Victory, OBE, MC, MBIM
Senior Scientific Officer	Miss Elisabeth Morse, MA, MSc

Table 2 (cont.)

Chairmen of Committees

Scientific Advisory Committee	Professor A. S. Truswell, MB, ChB, MD, FRCP, MFCM (Head of the Department of Food Science & Nutrition, Queen Elizabeth College, University of London)
Industrial Scientists Committee	Professor R. J. L. Allen, OBE, MSc, PhD (Group Research Director, Beecham Group Limited. Visiting Professor of Applied Nutrition at Guy's Hospital Medical School (University of London))
Information Committee	Gordon L. Shemilt, DFC (Director, Tate and Lyle Limited)
Editorial Advisory Board	Dr. Magnus Pyke, BSc, PhD, FRIC, FIBiol, FIFST, FRSE (Secretary, British Association for the Advancement of Science)

The Council and its Committees

Having explained the set-up as regards the Officers, I will now run through briefly the Council and its Committees which constitute the main machinery for the conduct of the Foundation's affairs.

The Council

(a) The Council consists of up to forty Governors — twenty Industrial Governors and twenty Scientific Governors. Here again, balance is maintained as with the rotation of the appointment of the Chairman and Vice-Chairman between an Industrialist and a Scientist.

(b) The Industrial Governors are all Directors of Member Companies though provision is made for the appointment of up to three Industrial Governors who need not be Directors of Members Companies but are eminent in business or industry.

(c) The Scientific Governors are, in the words of our Articles of Association, "scientists of repute in their particular fields but not in the employment of Member Companies". Consequently they are all academic scientists drawn from universities, research institutes, government departments and other bodies. At the pre sent time eight of them are medically qualified. Included in the twenty Scientific Governors are two who are appointed by the Royal Society of London.

(d) The Council meets four times a year and deals with all policy, membership and financial matters. They appoint a small Executive Committee of eight members to whom they delegate full powers other than final approval of the annual budget.

The Scientific Advisory Committee

(a) The Scientific Advisory Committee consists of not more than twenty-four persons who are scientists or educationalists of repute in their particular fields but are not in the employment of any Member Company. In addition, the President, Chairman, Vice-Chairman, Honorary Treasurer and Director-General are *ex-officio* members of the Committee.

(b) The Committee is responsible for making recommendations to the Council as to suitable fields in which the Foundation might carry out, or advance, promote or procure the carrying out of research and investigation, and as to suitable persons, corporations or institutions to which the Foundation might give pecuniary or other help.

(c) The Committee is appointed annually by the Council.

The Industrial Scientists Committee

(a) This Committee consists of not more than twenty-four persons who are senior scientists in full-time employment of Member Companies.

(b) The Committee is responsible for:

(i) giving advice and assistance to the Scientific Advisory Committee on any matter which the Scientific Advisory Committee should so request;

(ii) bringing to the notice of the Scientific Advisory Committee and, where appropriate, the Council, scientific developments in the processing, manufacture and storage of food and to make recommendations where such developments appear to merit the establishment of an *ad hoc* committee for specific studies.

(c) Members of the Committee are appointed annually by the Council.

The Information Committee

(a) This Committee consists of not more than fifteen persons who have experience in public relations, formal education, or in communication with other organizations and members of the public.

(b) The specific duties of the Committee are:

(i) monitoring the activities of the Public Relations Consultants retained by the Foundation;

(ii) generally supervising and keeping in touch with the flow of information from the Foundation to Member Companies, other organizations and members of the public;

(iii) advising, and making recommendations to, the Council on all matters connected with education and the flow of information.

(c) As with the other Committees, Members are appointed annually by the Council.

The Editorial Advisory Board

(a) This Board has recently been reorganized and enlarged and now consists of twenty-eight persons who have experience in education, publication or communication by the written word with other organizations and with members of the public.

(b) The Board never meets as such but individual members are asked to comment on and referee proposed articles for our *Nutrition Bulletin* which are in their particular sphere of interest.

(c) The Board has an Executive Committee which meets twice a year with the main purpose of approving articles for, and making policy decisions on, our *Nutrition Bulletin*. This Executive Committee consists of six persons but, in addition, the President, Chairman, Vice-Chairman and Director-General are *ex-officio* members.

(d) The Board is elected annually by the Council and its specific duties are:

  (i) advising, and making recommendations to, the Council on all matters connected with the BNF *Nutrition Bulletin;*

  (ii) deciding as to the material to be included in the *Bulletin;*

  (iii) as required, advising and making recommendations to the Council on all matters relating to BNF publications.

So much for the organization of the Foundation. I would now like to tell you something of our work in:

(a) support for Research,

(b) dissemination of Information,

(c) encouragement of Education.

Support for Research

Early Days

During the early years the emphasis in the Foundation's activities was on support for Research. In this the Scientific Advisory Committee played a leading role in that it studied the many applications for grants which were received, assessed their relevance to the work of the Foundation in nutritional matters, and made recommendations to the Council on the merits of grant applications. Final power to allocate grants was vested only in the Council.

Types of Grants

Grants were made to promote research in nutritional matters through the payment of salaries, the purchase of capital equipment or expendable supplies and, exceptionally, to support scientific meetings. Consideration was also given to providing travel and related expenses to enable younger scientists to contribute to meetings abroad.

By early 1972 a pattern in the nature of grant applications had developed and the Council decided to review its policy with the object of ensuring that the best possible use was made of the limited funds available for the support of Research. As a result of this the Council decided on the following five priority areas for the allocation of research grants:

(a) Energy requirements.
(b) Fibre.
(c) Genetic factors in nutrition.
(d) Obesity.
(e) Role of gut flora in human nutrition.

In May 1975 the Council again reviewed its policy on the allocation of funds as between Research, Information and Education and a major decision was taken. However, I will have more to say on this later.

Research Conference

In pursuance of its policy at the time of affording priority to Research, the Council decided to hold a Research Conference at Churchill College, Cambridge, in April 1973. Attendance was by invitation, the Foundation paying all travel and accommodation expenses, and there were some 115 people, mainly scientists, present.

There were many distinguished speakers, including some from overseas, and the proceedings of the conference were published in a book entitled *Nutritional Problems in a Changing World* [1] within 6 months of the conference being held. Since then, about 1700 copies of the book have been sold and it is likely to be reprinted.

Some Projects Supported

During the period 1970-1976 the Foundation allocated about £128,000 in support of Research. Many projects were supported and you may be interested to hear of just a few of them:

(a) Peptide absorption and its nutritional importance.

(b) Intestinal absorption in the elderly.

(c) Nutritional control of toxicity.

(d) Role of the gut flora in the metabolism of food additives, drugs and toxic agents.

(e) Studies in fat absorption.

(f) Endocrines and bodyweight.

(g) Dietary fibre and its influence on bile acid metabolism.

(h) The effect of diet on hydroxylation of benzpyrene and nitrosamines in lung and kidney.

(i) The regulation of energy balance on obesity.

All grantees are required to produce reports on their work and summaries of these appear each year in our Annual Report.

Before leaving Research I must mention one major grant we have made towards nutritional education in universities. In 1972 we established a lectureship at the University of Leeds. The newly appointed lecturer took responsibility for the new Food Science/Physiology combined studies BSc degree course at the University. He was also in a position to strengthen research on nutrition in the Department of Physiology and to assist in the general growth of nutritional studies in the University and in the Leeds area. I am happy to say that after our initial grant of £10,000 to establish the lectureship, subsequent financial responsibility for maintaining it was accepted by the University.

Dissemination of Information

Early Development

While the early support for Research was in full swing, work on the dissemination of information steadily developed. A major step forward in this direction was taken in mid-1972 by adding to the Staff a Scientific Information Officer—now known as the Senior Scientific Officer because the responsibilities of the post have rapidly expanded and developed since the first appointment was made.

In addition to this, in January 1973 the Council appointed a Public Relations Consultancy to take over from the Public Relations Officer who had hitherto been retained on a part-time basis. Their primary task was to advise and assist the Foundation in disseminating the considerable amount of Information it had to offer, and to develop and expand the contacts with the media which had already been made by the Permanent Officers.

It was from this time on that the Foundation's work in Information really took hold and as the Foundation became better known amongst the media, and throughout the country in general, so the demands on it for the provision of more and more Information grew.

Relations with the Media and Other Bodies

As far as the media are concerned, the position is now well established. They frequently consult us and we hold occasional informal buffet lunches for small groups of up to six journalists, the objects of which are to hear their views and problems, and to put over to them our latest thoughts on selected matters. In addition to this, over the past few years the Director-General and the Senior Scientific Officer have been asked to make an increasing number of radio and TV broadcasts on nutritional matters.

We now hold two or three Press Conferences a year and these are usually connected with making major comments on some topical nutritional matters or launching publications. We have learnt that it is very important to be able to work closely with the media but we have also come to recognize that this is sometimes not without its hazards. For example, after Press Conferences some journalists might report on only one aspect of a point that has been made, because they consider it to be newsworthy, rather than giving the overall balanced picture which we always aim to put over on such occasions.

In pursuance of our work in Information, we maintain close contact with other "opinion-formers", such as consumer groups and similar bodies, and we also receive several requests for information from members of the public.

Publications

Expansion of our work in Information inevitably led to publications. Apart from our *Nutrition Bulletin,* the three major publications we have made over the past few years have been our two leaflets entitled "Healthy eating for the elderly" and "Healthy eating in pregnancy" and our most recent one is a substantial booklet called *Why Additives? — The Safety of Foods.*[2] Close on 50,000 copies of each of the two "Healthy eating" leaflets have now been sold and latest reports are that sales of the "Why Additives?" booklet are going very well indeed. It was certainly well received by the media. In addition to these, we have just published in conjunction with the Health Education Council two new leaflets entitled "Healthy eating for your children" and "the Overweight child" which will be distributed free.

Our only, but important, regular publication is our *Nutrition Bulletin.* This is published three times a year—in January, May and September—and from all the reports that come back to us, it is a highly regarded publication. Up until 2 years ago we used to distribute it free but the annual costs of so doing began to approach £5,000. Consequently, we decided to institute a modest subscription charge of £3 a year. Unfortunately this resulted in a worrying drop in circulation and we are currently examining ways and means of promoting sales.

Films

I must just mention two films in the production of which we played a leading role. The first was "In place of the sun" for which we met half the costs and produced in conjunction with what was then called the Community Relations Commission. It is a colour film in cartoon form and is designed to inform Asian immigrants of nutritional information important in the avoidance of rickets. The second film called "A way of life" was on obesity and we acted as scientific, treatment and script advisers. This film was, however, financed by the Health Education Council and the Scottish Health Education Unit. Both films were very well received and have enjoyed a high sales rate and a high lending rate from film libraries.

Second Conference

Finally under information, though it also extends to Research and Education, I would like to mention our second major conference which was again held at Churchill College, Cambridge, in April 1976. Unlike our first research conference, this second one had a distinct socio-economic slant and was entitled "People and Food Tomorrow" [3] which was a very topical theme. Although this conference was on a subscription basis it was very well supported and we again succeeded in having the book of proceedings published within 6 months. I am happy to say that sales of this book are also going very well.

Encouragement of Education

I would now like to say a few words about some of our work in Education. There is, of course, as you will appreciate, something of an overlap between Information and Education, and some of our activities I have referred to when discussing Information—particularly our publications and films—also have a bearing on Education.

In the interests of time, there are just three particular activities in Education I would like to refer to and they are:

(a) Seminars for Member Companies.

(b) Food and nutrition resources kit for teachers.

(c) Working Party on Nutrition Education.

Seminars for Member Companies

Two years ago, in 1975, we decided that it might be helpful to marketing executives of Member Companies if they had a better background knowledge of nutrition. We arranged a one day seminar for them entitled "Putting Nutrition to Work".

The seminar was organized on a self-financing basis and was very well attended. The ground covered included:

(a) Principles of human nutrition.

(b) Good health—role of nutrition.

(c) Maintaining maximum nutritional value in production and marketing.

(d) Food additives today.

(e) Nutritional labelling.

This seminar was such a success that in 1976 we held a second one designed for production managers entitled "Nutrition and Food Production". This was equally well supported, was much appreciated by those present, and the ground covered included the following:

(a) Some principles of human nutrition.

(b) Nutrients in foods.

(c) How nutrient requirements are met in Britain.

(d) Effects of processing, storage and cooking of foods on their nutrients.

(e) Consumer research and product development.

(f) Food standards and legislation.

(g) Nutritional labelling.

Food and Nutrition Resources Kit for Teachers

Over the years we have received many requests for information from teachers engaged in running food and nutrition courses in schools at all levels. We also received requests for information from students and school children who were undertaking a project in some aspects of nutrition.

A pattern of the information required quickly developed and consequently we decided to produce a "Food and nutrition resources kit" for teachers designed to cover the requirements. We sell this at the modest sum of £1.60 a kit and sales have increased encouragingly as the availability of the kit has become more widely known.

The kit is quite comprehensive and includes some of our own publications, extensive lists of books and pamphlets on various aspects of nutrition and food commodities, details of visual aids available including films, and notes on nutrition courses available throughout the country. When we send it out we invite comments from recipients as to what they would like to see included in the kit and we update it on a regular basis.

Working Party on Nutrition Education

When he was Secretary of State for Social Services in 1973, the Rt. Hon. Sir Keith Joseph, MP, was the Guest Speaker at our Annual Luncheon. In his speech, amongst other things, he discussed nutrition education and said he would like to see a working party set up by his Department and the Foundation with the task of examining the present state of nutrition education in the country and how it could be improved.

The Working Party was duly set up and comprised representatives of the Department of Health and Social Security, the British Nutrition Foundation and the Health Education Council. It proved to be a bigger task than was at first thought and it was only in the spring of 1977 that the Working Party completed their deliberations and produced their final report for the Secretary of State.

The report is now being printed and will be published by the Department of Health and Social Security within the next 2 months, hopefully with a Foreword by the Rt. Hon. David Ennals, MP, the present Secretary of State for Social Services.

The report makes some important recommendations and if these are finally accepted a somewhat enhanced role for the Foundation to play in nutrition education will emerge and we will have to step up considerably our activities in this area.

Present Policy

I would now like to say something about our present policy. As you can see from the review I have given you of our work in Research, Information and Education over the years, by early 1975 our activities in the latter two spheres had increased very considerably and all this had been achieved without any increases in staff.

In May 1975 the Council decided to review their policy on the allocation of resources as between Research, Information and Education. By then the Agricultural Research Council/Medical Research Council (ARC/MRC) Report on Food and Nutrition Research (the Neuberger Report) [4] had been published. Some of you will no doubt have had the opportunity to read this report. The Council warmly welcomed the report and agreed with the recommendations as to the areas of research with special importance or urgency. However, the cost of Research was becoming increasingly high and the Foundation had by then allocated some £120,000 in support of Research which had been somewhat of a strain on its resources.

After some deliberation the Council decided that the time had come to change direction as far as support for Research was concerned and concluded that in the future, for the time being anyway, the Foundation had an important role to play in social nutrition and that every effort should be made to interpret and disseminate the results of Research in this and other areas through the mediums of Information and Education.

In May 1975 the Council announced its new policy which can be summarized as follows:

(a) The Foundation's support for Research will be redirected towards "pump-priming" projects, including social nutrition. Priority will be given to young scientists embarking on postgraduate work in nutrition and the medical students' prize will continue.

(b) Activities relating to the dissemination of nutritional information and the encouragement of education in nutrition will continue to be expanded.

One last point on this. You will notice mention is made of the medical students' prize and perhaps you might like to know the background. About 5 years ago we became concerned about the lack of nutritional education for medical students and so we set up an annual prize essay competition. Students are required to write an essay on any aspect of nutrition of their choosing. The winner is awarded a grant of £500 to enable him, or her, to spend up to 3 months of an elective period in a developing country studying some specific aspect of under-nutrition. All the prize-winners have done good work and reports on their projects have appeared in our *Nutrition Bulletin*.

Membership of the Foundation

Having reviewed our organization and activities you may now be interested to hear something about membership of the Foundation. Originally membership was open only to companies engaged in the food, drink and allied industries. However, 3 years ago our Articles of Association were amended and as a result of this all Scientific Governors became members of the Foundation in their own individual right but without financial commitment.

We now have forty-four Member Companies. They include nearly all the major food-manufacturing companies, some of the large retailers and several smaller companies. The basic annual subscription to the Foundation to secure membership is £300. However, in addition to this, all the medium-sized and large companies make additional contributions in the form of either a 7-year Deed of Covenant or an Annual Donation guaranteed for a minimum period of 3 years.

Hitherto new Member Companies have been recruited mostly by individual Industrial Governors persuading their friends in other companies to join. Some of the Industrial Governors have been particularly successful at this and we have much to thank them for. Towards the end of this year we will be launching a major recruiting campaign and we all hope that the general economic situation in the country by then will enable us to be successful in this.

Our present annual budget is about £100,000. We are just getting through on this but if we are really to develop and expand our work in Research, Information and Education—particularly the latter two—we need about £160,000 and we are hoping that our forthcoming recruiting campaign will produce this. There is also the possibility that we may receive a grant from the Government to expand our work in Education following publication of the Report of the Working Party on Nutrition Education. However, this is conjectural at the moment and we cannot count on it.

Conclusion

Wherever money to support our activities comes from, there is one matter on which the Council is adamant—and that is that we must retain our position as a totally independent body. We are not a front for the food industry and nor must we become a tool of the Government. We must retain our ability to speak the truth on all nutritional matters, however much this might not be entirely agreeable to some interests.

We place particular importance on our liaison with other national nutrition foundations and we are always keen to develop this to the mutual benefit of all concerned. As practical evidence of this we like to play to the full our part in the Nutrition Foundation's Award Book Scheme. It gave us all particular pleasure to agree this year that an award should be made for that excellent publication—*Food: the Gift of Osiris.* [5] Although I know it caused him some embarrassment, I would like to say that we were particularly pleased that Professor William J. Darby of the Nutrition Foundation Inc., should have been one of the three co-authors. He has done so much to further the co-operation between the national nutrition foundations.

A major subject which is being studied by our Council and its committees at present is the role to be played should a National Food and Nutrition Policy be developed in the United Kingdom. There is talk of the possibility of this in some circles and we in the Foundation want to ensure that we are in on things from the outset and play our full part in influencing trends.

Finally, I would like to say that in the short time available it has only been possible for me to mention some of our work in Research, Information and Education. Much is going on all the time and we are doing our best to meet the many demands made on us. We are all spurred on by the thought that morale is high and we are all looking forward eagerly to meeting the increasing challenges which are coming our way.

I should like to acknowledge the great help I have received from the Foundation's Secretary, Mr. P. M. Victory, in the preparation of this Report.

References

1. *Nutritional Problems in a Changing World* (Proceedings of the BNF Research Conference 1973), edited by Dorothy Hollingsworth and Margaret Russell, Applied Science Publishers, 1973.

2. *Why Additives? - The Safety of Foods,* devised and edited by The British Nutrition Foundation, Forbes Publications Ltd., 1977.

3. *People and Food Tomorrow* (Proceedings of the Second BNF Conference 1976), edited by Dorothy Hollingsworth and Elisabeth Morse. Applied Science Publishers, 1976.

4. Agricultural Research Council/Medical Research Council, 1974, *Food and Nutrition Research,* Report by the ARC/MRC Committee, London, HMSO.

5. William J. Darby, Paul Ghalioungui and Louis Grivetti, 1977, *Food: The Gift of Osiris,* Academic Press Inc. (London) Ltd.

Nutrition Research in Switzerland

J. C. Somogyi

Director, Institute for Nutrition Research, Rüschlikon-Zürich

I shall try to give an overview on nutrition research in Switzerland and some details on the work of my Institute, followed by a brief information on nutrition education in our country. I can restrict myself to certain points because of Professor Aebi's contribution on the promotion of nutrition research in Switzerland.

May I mention that in Switzerland we have only one institute which deals exclusively with problems of human nutrition. This is the Institute for Nutrition Research in Rüschlikon-Zürich, which I direct. However, there are several laboratories at various universities and in industry, in which individual research workers or research groups are concerned with nutritional problems.

Within the Swiss Federal Institute of Technology, an institution which is comparable to the MIT in Boston, there exists an Institute for Animal Nutrition which carries out investigations mainly on energy metabolism of domestic animals and on various problems pertaining to meat and fats, of which experiments on the toxic factors in rapeseed oil appear to be rather important.

Reverting to human nutrition a pioneer survey of Professor Verzar and Dr. Schlettwein-Gsell on the nutrition and health status of the Swiss population, with particular reference to the situation of the farmers in the mountainous part of the country, has to be quoted. The results of this investigation, which lasted several years, were published in book form in 1962.[1] Following this survey, Dr. Schlettwein-Gsell from the University of Basle has specialized in epidemiological investigations, on the nutritional status of certain groups of the Swiss population in different regions of the country. These surveys are valuable contributions in this field.[2,3]

Interesting investigations were performed by Professor Ritzel and Professor Brubacher respectively, both from Basle, on the vitamin, mainly the thiamine status of students, elderly people, etc. These studies[4,5] show, for example, that students as well as elderly people have a suboptimal supply of this vitamin. Professor Ritzel has recently published another interesting study on the social factors of obesity in children.[6]

The Department of Vitamin and Nutrition Research of the Hoffmann La Roche Company is also active in nutrition research, particularly in the assessment of the vitamin status in humans and the determination of vitamins in food. This department has developed amongst others a method for the assessment of vitamin B_2 by the determination of the glutathion reductase in red blood cells or whole blood.[7] Professor Brubacher, Dr. Vuilleumier and other members of this department are very cooperative and always willing to help other research groups engaged in similar investigations.

In this connection the so-called Basler Study by Widmer and co-workers[8] has to be mentioned; it was carried out on about 6400 employees and workers of the chemical industries in Basle. This survey was originally planned as a prospective study on the risk factors of heart and vascular diseases of atherosclerotic origin. In a later phase, however, the relationship between the nutritional status and coronary heart disease has also been investigated.[9]

Important research on nutrition is performed also in the Research Laboratories of the Nestlé Company. This work is mainly concerned with various protein problems.[10,11] Head of this Group is Professor Mauron, who is teaching nutrition at the University of Fribourg. I do not speak about the activities of the Nestlé Foundation because Professor Aebi, its vice-president, can give more detailed information.

Obesity has been studied experimentally as well as clinically by Professor Renold and his co-workers[12] by Professor Jeaneraud,[13] both in Geneva, and Professor Stauffacher[14] in Basle. Professor Hartmann[15] from Chur has carried out investigations on the relationship between obesity and physical exercise.

Professor Aebi of the University of Bern has been interested for many years in nutrition. His investigations on vitamin D are well known. He conducts at present very interesting experiments on the influence of nutritional factors in the regulation of enzyme activity. He was the initiator of the Foundation for the Promotion of Nutrition Research in Switzerland (Stiftung zur Förderung der Ernährungsforschung in der Schweiz), which plays an important role in the promotion of nutrition research and of nutrition training of young Swiss scientists.

Interesting surveys have been performed on the nutritional value of food in elderly people's homes, on food habits of adolescents[16] and on the epidemiology of atherosclerosis[17] by the Institute of Social and Preventive Medicine in Zürich under the direction of Professor Schär.

The Department of Caries Research of the University of Zürich is also involved in nutrition problems. This group under Professor Mühlemann has carried out experiments on the inhibition of the solubility of enamel by various fluorine compounds. In this field I co-operated with him for many years.[18,19]

Furthermore, his group has studied the pH changes of microbial plaque after the intake of different nutrients by pH telemetry. They developed a special apparatus for the wireless measurement of pH, whereby a mini-transmitter was placed and fixed in the mouth of the probands. The pH telemetry facilitated the clarification of the acidogenicity of various nutrients, especially of various carbohydrates, to a great extent. This method is used for the "official" testing of so-called "sweets safe for teeth".

Interesting epidemiological investigations were performed by Professor Marthaler and Dr. Regolati[20,21] on the effect of fluoridated table salt on the caries incidence of children and adolescents. Their study shows a significant reduction of caries after 3-5 years use of salt containing 250 mg NaF/kg.

About 3 years ago the Institute of Food Science was formed by the fusion of the Department of Agricultural Chemistry, the Department of Dairy Sciences, and the Department of Food Processing and Technology at the Swiss Federal Institute of Technology in Zürich. This institute was completed later by the addition of a Department of Food Microbiology.

Finally I would like to deal with the work of our Institute. This was founded in 1958 and is sponsored to the greatest part by the Green Meadow Foundation and partly by grants from the Federal Government. The connection with the University is close, since I teach nutrition to medical students and, on the other hand, we co-operate with several institutes and clinics.

In these past 19 years our investigations have been conducted in a biochemical as well as in an epidemiological direction. The most important ones can be summarized as follows:

For many years we have worked on the elucidation of the chemical structure of naturally occurring antagonists of thiamine. These antithiamine factors—as I designated them—are present among others in the viscera of various species of fish, predominantly in intestines of carps and in plants, e.g. in bracken fern. These antithiamines play a role in the nutrition of domestic animals and can be of importance in human nutrition as well.[22]

The opinions on the chemical nature of these compounds have been conflicting for a long time, because they had not been isolated in a pure state. Our work concentrated on this aspect. My group could establish that a thermostable antithiamine factor contained in carp viscera in a hemin-derivative (Kündig and Somogyi[23]). Later Berüter and myself[24] isolated an antithiamine factor from bracken fern. This was identified as 3,4-dihydroxy cinnamic acid, i.e. caffeic acid. As shown by the investigations of Bönicke and Somogyi,[25] similar inactivation is brought about by various *o*-dihydroxy phenols. By determinating the urinary thiamine excretion we recently could demonstrate that these *o*-diphenols possess an antithiamine effect also in humans.[26] Vimokesant and co-workers[27] in Bangkok made similar observations on the antithiamine effects of tea and of some habitual foods in man—all containing these *o*-dihydroxy phenols.[28]

Other experiments dealt with the biosynthesis of ascorbic acid in potatoes,[29,30] with the sucrose, glucose and fructose contents of various fruits and vegetables,[31,32] whereby these sugars were determined enzymatically. These latter investigations have found considerable interest among the diabetologists, the specialists in internal medicine, as well as the practitioners.

The investigations on changes of the sucrose-. glucose-, fructose-, and vitamin C content of various fruits during ripening were recently terminated (Somogyi and Trautner[33]).

A great number of our experiments and of our publications deal with the nutritional value of potatoes, with the changes of their vitamin C and B_1 content due to storage, household and industrial handling.[34,35,36]

In this connection should be mentioned that my group is generally interested in the changes and losses of nutrients, especially of vitamins caused by household and industrial handling. The results of our investigations on this topic have been published in several papers.[37,38]

Another problem with which we dealt was food irradiation. In cooperation with the Federal Research Institute for Fruit Growing and Viniculture, Wädenswil—Zürich, we investigated whether and under what conditions the storage time of fruits and vegetables between harvest and distribution can be prolonged by gamma-irradiation. Simultaneously the changes in the contents of vitamin C and of various sugars were determined.

Further experiments have shown that irradiation of potatoes causes a pronounced, about 8-10-fold, increase of sucrose.[39] This rise is connected—as our very recent experiments reveal—with a simultaneous increase of the activities of phosphorylase and saccharose synthetase.[40]

For several years we have been working on the assessment of the thiamine and niacin status and, since this past year, also on the iron status in humans. The methods for the assessment of the thiamine and niacin status have been improved.

The following epidemiological surveys were performed by our group:

1. About the eating and drinking habits of students (650 persons) of our university.[41]

2. On the nutritional, especially on the thiamine status of healthy persons, chronic alcoholics and former alcoholics.[42,43,44] We also have for a long time investigated the relationship between alcohol and nutrition. Chronic alcoholism not only causes deterioration of the nutritional status, but, in addition, the food composition has repercussions on alcohol consumption as, among others, our experiments with rats, carried out together with Professor Bättig[45] have demonstrated. Similar investiga-

tions with humans have just started.

3. On the nutritional status of elderly people, who prepare their own meals (keep their own household).

4. Another study was done in co-operation with Professor Schär and co-worker on the nutrient content of meals from the canteens of the University of Zürich and the Swiss Federal Institute of Technology.[46]

Our investigations, in which the niacin status of students and elderly people was compared, yielded interesting results. In particular, we have observed that after oral niacinamide intake the urinary excretion of the metabolites *N'*-methylnicotinamide and *N'*-methyl-2-pyridone-5-carboxylamide seems to be more rapid than after nicotinic acid administration.[47]

Some other subjects with which we have dealt are: communal feeding, nutrition and atherosclerosis, the relationship between nutrition and dental caries.

The Institute organizes regularly international symposia, in a few instances also in co-operation with other scientific organizations, e.g. the Group of European Nutritionists. The most important meetings are listed in Table 1.

The proceedings of these symposia, as well as of the meetings of the Group of European Nutritionists, appear in the series of our publications, in the Bibliotheca *Nutritio et Dieta,* of which 25 volumes have been published until now (Table 2).

Finally, a few words on *nutrition education of the public.* This task lays mainly in the hands of the Swiss Association for Nutrition which was founded in 1966 and which, with about 4300 members, is one of the largest organizations of this kind in Europe. The unusually rapid growth of the Association shows the great interest of the Swiss population for nutritional problems; it was facilitated by the support of a governmental agency which provides rooms and staff for the secretariat of the Association.

According to the Statutes, the Association should promote the contact between science and practice. In fact, the members are recruited from scientists, nutritionists, physicians, dentists, dieticians, home economists, interested laymen, etc. The Association in general organizes two meetings on nutritional problems annually (Table 3, and acts as the publisher of a series of booklets on nutrition aimed at the general public.

We have in Switzerland another society in this field. This is the Swiss Society for Nutrition Research, whose members are exclusively scientists working in the area of nutrition. An excellent co-operation exists between these two societies.

I hope that this paper—even though a selection of this kind of course is always subjective—has given an insight into the various activities taking place in the field of nutrition research in Switzerland.

Table 1

Symposia and meetings of the Institute for Nutrition Research

Modern Problems of Nutrition
organized on the occasion of the opening of the Institute for Nutrition Research
Rüschlikon, 18th April 1959

Well-balanced Nutrition and Communal Feeding
joint meeting of the Institute for Nutrition Research, the Swiss Society for Nutrition Research and the Swiss Association for Preventive Medicine
Baden, 12th-13th May 1960

Nutrition Science in the Service of Developing Countries
Zürich and Feldbach, 18th-20th October 1961

Connection Between Nutrition and Dental Caries
Zürich, 16th-18th October 1962

Antivitamins
Zürich and Feldbach, 19th-21st October 1964

Changes in Foods Due to Industrial Handling
Rüschlikon, 26th March 1965

Food Irradiation—Present Status and Future Possibilities
under the patronage of the Federal Commission for Food Irradiation
Zürich, 7th April 1967

Nutrition and Atherosclerosis
symposium and postgraduate course for physicians
Bad Ragaz, 24th-26th October 1968

Biological interrelations and nutrition
organized in co-operation with the Group of European Nutritionists on the occasion of the 10th anniversary of the Institute for Nutrition Research
Zürich and Feldbach, 15th-18th April 1969

Table 1 (cont.)

The Challenge of Synthetic and Substitute Foods
joint meeting with the Gottlieb Duttweiler Institute for Economic and Social Studies
Rüschlikon, 5th-6th February 1970

Nutrition Research and Food Production
Zürich, 9th-10th April 1970

Newer Knowledge on the Connection Between Nutrition and Dental Health
presentation of the Gottlieb Duttweiler Prize for the promotion of nutritional sciences to Professor Dr. F. Bramstedt, Würzburg
Rüschlikon, 21st November 1970

Nutrition and Technology of Foods for Growing Humans
conference in co-operation with the International Union of Nutritional Sciences and with the International Union of Food Science and Technology
Zürich, 13th-15th October 1971

From Vitamin to Hormone: the Story of Vitamin D
presentation of the Gottlieb Duttweiler Prize for the promotion of nutritional sciences to Dr. E. Kodicek, Cambridge
Rapperswil, 23rd October 1972

Future Trends in Nutrition and Dietetics
Zürich and Feldbach, 29th-30th March 1973

Nutrition and Alcoholism
under the patronage of the Swiss Association for Nutrition
Zürich, 17th-18th October 1974

The Relationship Between the Frequency of Food Intake and Energy Metabolism
presentation of the Gottlieb Duttweiler Prize for the promotion of nutritional sciences to Dr. P. Fabry, Prague
Rapperswil, 25th November 1975

Nutritional, Psychological and Social Aspects of Obesity
joint meeting with the Group of European Nutritionists
Zürich, 8th-9th September 1976

Table 2

Bibliotheca Nutritio et Dieta
Series published by the Institute for Nutrition Research

Vol.	1.	Modern problems of nutrition. I	1960
Vol.	2.	Well-balanced nutrition and communal feeding	1961
Vol.	3.	Modern problems of nutrition. II	1962
Vol.	4.	Nutrition science in the service of developing countries	1962
Vol.	5.	Relationship between nutrition and dental caries	1963

Table 2 (cont.)

Vol. 6.	Nutrition and cardiovascular diseases	1964
Vol. 7.	The influence of industrial and household handling on the composition of food	1965
Vol. 8.	Antivitamins	1966
Vol. 9.	Minor constituents in foods	1967
Vol. 10.	Antibiotics in agriculture	1968
Vol. 11.	The influence of nutrition on the intermediary metabolism	1969
Vol. 12.	Nutrition and atherosclerosis	1969
Vol. 13.	Nutritional aspects of the development of bone and connective tissue	1969
Vol. 14.	Malnutrition is a problem of ecology	1970
Vol. 15.	Biological interrelations and nutrition	1970
Vol. 16.	Nutrition research and food production	1971
Vol. 17.	Nutrition and nervous system	1972
Vol. 18.	Nutrition and technology of foods for growing humans	1973
Vol. 19.	Clinical nutrition	1973
Vol. 20.	Assessment of nutritional status and food consumption survey	1974
Vol. 21.	Future trends in nutrition and dietetics	1975
Vol. 22.	The gut and nutrition	1975
Vol. 23.	Early signs of nutritional deficiencies	1976
Vol. 24.	Nutrition and alcoholism	1976
Vol. 25.	Nutritional aspects of fats	1977
Vol. 26.	Nutritional, psychological and social aspects of obesity	1978

Table 3

Meetings organized by the Swiss Association for Nutrition

The importance of nutritional science for public health
Zürich, 4th May 1966

Vitamins: the mode of their action and their significance for human health
Solothurn, 17th November 1966

How can man adapt his nutrition to the conditions of life in the technological age?
Present knowledge on the relationship between nutrition and dental health
Bern, 19th May 1967

Table 3 (cont.)

Prevention of diabetes by diet Basel, 27th October 1967
The importance of fats in nutrition. Modern ways of the production of fats and oils Luzern, 9th May 1968
The importance of fruits, vegetables and potatoes in our nutrition. New ways and means of the industrial utilization of fruit Weinfelden, 21st September 1968
Nutrition and obesity. -The problem of overfeeding, especially of adolescents Biel, 30th May 1969
Nutrition, iron deficiency and anemia. - Protein malnutrition and the exploitation of new protein sources Lausanne, 27th November 1970
Lack and deficiencies in nutrition. - The role of calcium in health and disease Bern, 5th May 1971
Diet and dental hygiene in the South Pacific in comparison to Switzerland. - Changes in dietetics due to medical progress Freiburg, 27th January 1972
Nutrition and atherosclerosis. - Psychological aspects of nutrition Locarno-Muralto, 27th October 1972
Food habits and nutrition education. - Trace elements and their importance in nutrition Basel, 21st November 1973
Various aspects of eating between meals Baden, 16th May 1974
Nutrition in different age groups Biel, 23rd May 1975
Critical remarks on various régimes for weight reduction Chur, 14th November 1975
Food additives - for or against health? Bern, 26th March 1976
Prevention of diseases by diet Lugano, 6th May 1977

Literature

1. Verzar, F. and Gsell, D. *Ernährung und Gesundheitszustand der Bergbevölkerung der Schweiz.* Eidg. Gesundheitsamt, Bern, 1962.

2. Schlettwein-Gsell, D., Bronsveld-Minder, B. and Ritzel, G. Nahrungskonsum von 1088 Jugendlichen in Basel. *Z. Präventivmedizin,* **18,** 269-277 (1973).

3. Schlettwein-Gsell, D. Erhebungen über die Ernährung von alten Menschen. im Buch: *Zur Ernährungssituation der schweizerischen Bevölkerung,* pp. 83-98 (Huber, Bern, 1975).

4. Ritzel, G. Untersuchungen über den Thiaminstatus einer schweizerischen Stadtbevölkerung. *Schweiz. Med. Wschr.* **98,** 1118-1121 (1968).

5. Brubacher, G., Haenel, A. and Ritzel, G. Zur Thiaminversorgung eines städtischen Kollektivs von Studenten. *Int. Z. Vit.-Ern. Forschung,* **42**, 451-456 (1972).

6. Ritzel, G. and Bückert, A. Sozialmedizinische Aspekte der Fettsucht. *Bibl. Nutr. Dieta,* **26,** 135-145 (Karger, Basel, 1978).

7. Glatzle, D., Körner, W. F., Christeller, S. and Wiss, O. Method for the detection of a biochemical riboflavin deficiency stimulation of $NADPH_2$-dependent glutathione reductase from human erythrocytes by FAD *in vitro* investigations on the vitamin B_2 status in healthy people and geriatric patients. *Int. J. Vit. Res.* **40,** 166-183 (1970).

8. Widmer, L. K., Kaufmann, L., Hartmann, G., Reber, H., Breil, H., Küng, H.-L., Pletscher, W., Schalch, W. R. and Buess, H. Organisation der Basler Studie über Arterien-, Venen- und Herzkrankheiten. *Schweiz. Med. Wschr.* **97,** 99-102 (1967).

9. Ritzel, G. Evaluation von Ernährungserhebungen im Rahmen der Basler Studie III. im Buch *Zur Ernährungssituation der schweizerischen Bevölkerung,* pp. 57-82 (Huber, Bern, 1975).

10. Mauron, J. Technology of protein synthesis and protein-rich foods. *Bibl. Nutr. Dieta,* **18,** 24-44 (Karger, Basel, 1973).

11. Antener, I., Verwilghen, A. M., Geert, C. van and Mauron, J. Dietary treatment of malnutrition balance-sheets of the main nutrients. Part II. *Int. J. Vit. Res.* **47,** 167-199 (1977).

12. Renold, A. E. and Cahill, G. F. Adipose tissue, in *Handbook of Physiology* No. 5 (Amer. Physiol. Soc., Washington, D.C., 1965a).

13. Jeanrenaud, B. and Hepp, D. Adipose tissue. Regulation and metabolic functions. *Horm. Metab. Res.* Suppl. 2 (Thieme, Stuttgart, 1970).

14. Stauffacher, W. Experimentelle Grundlagen der Fettsucht. *Bibl. Nutr. Dieta,* **16,** 1-6 (Karger, Basel, 1971).

15. Hartmann, G. Körperliche Aktivität und Uebergewicht. *Bibl. Nutr. Dieta,* **26,** 103-110 (Karger, Basel, 1978).

16. Stransky, M. and Schär, M. Gemeinschaftsverpflegung von Betagten und Jugendlichen in Zürich. im Buch: *Zur Ernährungssituation der schweizerischen Bevölkerung,* pp. 129-147 (Huber, Bern, 1975).

17. Stransky, M. Erziehungs- und Ernährungsstudie zur Verminderung des Herzinfarktrisikos. *Sozial- und Präventivmedizin,* **22,** 180-181 (1977).

18. Mühlemann, H. R., Somogyi, J. C. and Poretti, G. G. Uptake of fluorine on the crown surface of human teeth after different storage times. *Schweiz. Monatsschr. Zahnheilk.* **65,** 685- (1955).

19. Somogyi, J. C. and Mühlemann, H. R. Kalzium- und Phosphorabgabe des intakten Schmelzes Menschlicher Zähne unter verschiedenen Versuchsbedingungen. *Int. Z. Vitaminforsch.* **27,** 72-84 (1956).

20. Marthaler, T. M., Crousaz, Ph. de, Meyer, R., Regolati, B. and Robert, A. Der Kariesbefall im Kanton Waadt nach Umstellung von der Tablettenfluoridierung auf die Salzfluoridierung. *Sozial- und Präventivmedizin,* **20,** 255-261 (1975).

21. Regolati, B. Erfolge der zahnmedizinischen Prophylaxe in der Schweiz. *Sozial- und Präventivmedizin,* **20,** 279-283 (1975).

22. Somogyi, J. C. and Trautner, K. Die Antivitamine. in *Fermente*

Hormone—Vitamine, Band III/1, 140 Seiten (Thieme, Stuttgart, 1974).

23. Kündig, H. and Somogyi, J. C. Isolation of the active moiety of the antithiamine compound from carp viscera. *Int. Z. Vitaminforsch.* **37,** 476-481 (1967).

24. Berüter, J. and Somogyi, J. C. 3,4-Dihydroxycinnamic acid, an antithiamine factor of fern. *Experientia,* **23,** 996 (1967).

25. Somogyi, J. C. and Bönicke, R. Connection between chemical structure and antithiamine activity of various phenol derivatives. *Int. Z. Vitaminforsch.* **39,** 65-73 (1969).

26. Somogyi, J. C. and Nägeli, U. Antithiamine effect of coffee. *Int. J. Vit. Nutr. Res.* **46,** 149-153 (1976).

27. Vimokesant, S. L., Nakornchai, S., Dhanamitta, S. and Hilker, D. M. Effect of tea consumption in thiamine status in man. *Nutr. Reports Internat.* **9,** 371- (1974).

28. Vimokesant, S., Nimitmongkol, N., Phuwastien, P., Nakornchai, S., Sripojanart, S., Dhanamitta, S. and Hilker, D. M. Occurrence of neuropathies and anti-thiamine factors in food. *Proc. 9th Int. Congr. Nutrition Mexico 1972,* vol. 2, 251-253 (Karger, Basel, 1975).

29. Trautner, K. and Somogyi, J. C. Biosynthese von Vitamin C in Kartoffelscheiben. *Int. Z. Vitaminforsch.* **34,** 433-435 (1964).

30. Trautner, K. and Somogyi, J. C. Biosynthese von Vitamin C in Kartoffelscheiben. *Nutr. Dieta,* **7,** 196-210 (1965).

31. Dako, D. Y., Trautner, K. and Somogyi, J. C. Der Glukose-, Fruktose- und Saccharosegehalt verschiedener Früchte. *Schweiz. Med. Wschr.* **100,** 897-903 (1970).

32. Somogyi, J. C. and Trautner, K. Der Glukose-, Fruktose- und Saccharosegehalt verschiedener Gemüsearten. *Schweiz. Med. Wschr.* **104,** 177-182 (1974).

33. Somogyi, J. C. and Trautner, K. Changes of the sucrose-,

glucose-, fructose- and vitamin C content of various fruits during ripening (in press, 1978).

34. Somogyi, J. C. Aenderungen des Vitamin C-Gehaltes von Kartoffeln unter verschiedenen Versuchsbedingungen. *Int. Z. Vitaminforsch.* **34,** 122-131 (1964).

35. Somogyi, J. C. and Schiele, K. Der Vitamin C-Gehalt verschiedener Kartoffelsorten und seine Abnahme während der Lagerung. *Int. Z. Vitaminforsch.* **36,** 337-359 (1966).

36. Somogyi, J. C., Trautner, K. and Kopp, P. M. Die Bedeutung der Kartoffelerzeugnisse in der heutigen Ernährung. *Bibl. Nutr. Dieta,* **16,** 140-154 (Karger, Basel, 1971).

37. Somogyi, J. C. Einfluss der Zubereitungsweise auf den Vitamin C-Gehalt von Kartoffeln und Gemüse. *Ernährungsumschau,* **22,** 42-45 (1975).

38. Somogyi, J. C. Some problems of the improvement of the nutritive quality of foods. *Proc. 8th Int. Congr. Nutrition, Prague 1969,* pp. 773-777 (*Excerpta Med. Int. Congr. Series* No. 213),

39. Somogyi, J. C., Kopp, P. M. and Trautner, K. Der Einfluss ionisierender Strahlen und Chemischer Keimhemmungsmittel auf Keimung, Zuckergehalt und Verarbeitungsqualität von Kartoffeln. *Mitt. Gebiete Lebensm. Hyg.* **66,** 117-140 (1975).

40. Becker, D. P. and Somogyi, J. C. Zum Wirkungsmechanismus des Saccharoseanstiegs in bestrahlten Kartoffeln. I. Zusammenhang zwischen dem Anstieg des Saccharosegehaltes und der Phosphorylaseaktivität nach Gammabestrahlung. *Mitt. Gebiete Lebensm. Hyg.* **68,** 409-418 (1977).

41. Somogyi, J. C. and Kopp, P. M. Erhebungen über Ernährungsgewohnheiten von Studenten. *Ernährungsumschau,* **22,** 195-200 (1975).

42. Somogyi, J. C. and Kopp, P. M. Alcohol and nutritional status. *Proc. 9th Int. Congr. Nutrition Mexico 1972,* **1,** 212-224 (Karger, Basel, 1975).

43. Somogyi, J. C. and Kopp, P. M. Alkoholismus und Ernährungsstatus. *Bibl. Nutr. Dieta,* **24,** 17-31 (Karger, Basel, 1976).

44. Somogyi, J. C. Ernährungsstatus chronischer Alkoholiker in der Schweiz. im Buch *Zur Ernährungssituation der schweizerischen Bevölkerung,* pp. 148-166 (Huber, Bern, 1975).

45. Bättig, K. and Somogyi, J. C. Der unterschiedliche Einfluss eines eiweissreichen, eines kohlenhydratreichen und eines fettreichen Futters auf die spontane Alkoholpräferenz der Ratte. *Bibl. Nutr. Dieta,* **24,** 94-99 (Karger, Basel, 1976).

46. Stransky, M., Schär, M., Kopp, P. M. and Somogyi, J. C. Untersuchungen über den Nähr- und Wirkstoffgehalt der Mahlzeiten der Mensen der Universität Zürich und der Eidg. Technischen Hochschule (ETH), Zürich. *Mitt. Gebiete Lebensm. Hyg.* **66,** 400-412 (1975).

47. Somogyi, J. C. and Schönhauser, E. On the intermediary metabolism of niacin and niacinamide (in press, 1978).

The Netherlands Nutrition Foundation

Joseph Hautvast

Secretary General NNF

The Netherlands Nutrition Foundation ("Nederlands Instituut voor Volksvoeding") was founded in 1919 and the first director was Professor Dr. Evert Cornelis van Leersum. He was a very active man, who did not limit his scientific activities to one job and in one place. Since he was a gastro-enterologist, he had a real interest in nutritional problems. His other interests were in the fields of Pharmacology and Medical History. He held chairs in the medical faculties of the Universities of Leyden, Utrecht and Amsterdam.

The Netherlands Nutrition Foundation was founded by Professor van Leersum himself. Under his guidance an institute was begun, specializing in nutrition research in the Netherlands. Reasons for doing this were as follows:

World War One had shown that nutritional knowledge was very important and necessary;

nutrition could play a role in national health and national development;

the science of nutrition in other countries had made some progress already.

Professor van Leersum had much financial support for his initiative, not only from governmental institutions, but also from many food industries. In the twenties much research was done on vitamins. After some years, however, the first signs of the general economic crisis were also felt by the Foundation and money for research became scarce. The end of the first prosperous period of the Netherlands Nutrition Foundation came in 1931, and the period from then until 1938 can be described as being a sort of "wintersleep".

Then a new period started, when Professor Dr. B. C. P. Jansen was appointed as the new director of the Foundation. Under the stimulating and active guidance of this eminent scientist, the objectives of the Foundation to promote nutritional and health research in general could be continued. His work, together with Donath in Indonesia, on the isolation of vitamin B_1 from rice polishings, had already made him world famous. He was father and leader of a first group of Netherlands nutritionists, who were trained in his laboratory. During his directorship of the Foundation, which lasted until 1956, he had close contacts with Charles Glen King, the Scientific Director of the Nutrition Foundation Inc. of the USA. Undoubtedly they discussed the activities of both Foundations and in a short review, published in 1954 in the Netherlands *Journal of Nutrition* ("Voeding"), Charles Glen King wrote about Professor B. C. P. Jansen.

After the retirement of Professor Jansen again a difficult period started. His successor in the University Department had no interest at all to continue the nutrition research. In 1959 the Foundation's research activities were moved from Amsterdam to the State Agricultural University in Wageningen. Here, the activities could become more closely linked with the most important basis of human nutrition, namely the Agricultural Sciences.

From 1961 the third period of progress started under the directorship of Professor Dr. Cornelis den Hartog, who held a chair in Human Nutrition in the Agricultural University. Close scientific links were established between the research activities of the Foundation and those of the Department of Human Nutrition of the Agricultural University. In the sixties good relations were established with the food industry and a large number of significant contributions in nutritional research were made. It would take too much time to give a complete review but one of those I would like to mention here is the participation in the international project on atherosclerosis, coordinated by Ancel Keys. However, at the end of the sixties it became more and more difficult to get nutritional research financed by either the food industry or Government.

In 1971 the Board of the Netherlands Nutrition Foundation decided to stop the Foundation's laboratory activities because the assignments for future research projects were considered to be too vague. The Board started the discussion on how to continue its work in the future in order to serve the objectives of the Foundation.

Now, in 1977, the Foundation has formulated its new objectives for the future and some of them are mentioned here.

1. An adaptation of the regulations of the Foundation will take place in 1977. It should be mentioned that there are at present no representatives from the food industry on the Board. This situation is most undesirable since the Foundation wants a good, though scientifically independent, relationship with the food industries. After discussion it was decided that the most favourable composition of the Board would be of twelve members: three of them representing the so-called "independent" people, a further three industrial members and the other six will be scientists ("expert members") who are involved in research and education activities in the field of human nutrition. The chairman should be appointed from the "independent" group, the treasurer from the "industrial" members and the secretary-general (executive officer) should be one of the "expert" members. The work of the Board will be supported by a small staff. At present two qualified people have a part-time appointment with the Foundation, each of them with a specific job description. The "industrial" members are going to represent the group of Trustees which will be set up and the same will occur for the nutrition expert members.

2. The financial resources of the Foundation at the moment are its own capital and some small donations, which it receives from industries and institutions. The capital was received in the past from food industries and is now for a great part invested. We are formulating the way in which regular financial support can be obtained from leading representatives of the food and allied industries.

In addition, the Foundation accepts, under certain conditions, money from food industries to be used for specific research work. It is the responsibility of the Foundation to contact researchers and to promote the research programme. This way of dealing with research programmes via our Foundation advances an independent relationship between food industry and researcher.

3. The following can be mentioned about the research activities of our Foundation.

Since 1974 we have supported a research programme on the role of bread in human nutrition. We have concentrated our interests on the sociological, psychological and behavioural aspects involved in the bread-eating, we chose this subject because we recognized that this kind of research will be of considerable importance in the future and by promoting such a study it will stimulate other research in this field.

Other research activities are limited to grants for PhD students, e.g. we have given some support for a study of food distribution in World War Two (1942-1944) in The Netherlands.

4. The Foundation strongly emphasizes the promoting of nutrition education programmes in the Universities. Since 1947 a "Netherlands Nutrition Foundation" chair has been accepted by the University of Amsterdam, a University with which the Foundation has a special relationship. The chair is in the Faculty of Biological Sciences and nutrition courses are given for students who want them. Students are given the opportunity to carry out nutritional research as part of their MSc degree course.

Recently the University of Amsterdam has asked the Board of the Foundation whether they would be willing to accept an extension of the teaching activities into the programme of the Medical Faculty of that University. This request will be discussed in the next meeting of our Board and, if the financial consequences of such an extension can be accepted, I am sure that the Board will favour this proposal. Within the same scope I can tell you about another decision, taken by the Board in the beginning of this year. It was decided that the Foundation should set up and take responsibility over, a second professorship in the field of human nutrition in a University and preferably in a medical faculty. We all know that nutrition education in medical training is very often neglected and this is also true for the Netherlands. In our country we have at present eight medical faculties and in only one of them (Leyden University) is there a chair in Human Nutrition. The Foundation wants to show its leadership in this field and considers initiative and support in this field as its task. Besides the promotion of nutrition education in universities the Foundation has also other education programmes on its list of activities. The most important one is that students, graduating for a degree in human nutrition, can receive small additional grants when performing special research work, like, for example, in developing countries.

The Netherlands Nutrition Foundation will, in all probability, take the lead in organizing post graduate courses in human nutrition for medical people. A preliminary date for starting these courses is September 1978, depending on the availability of teaching and administrative personnel and financial resources.

5. Another activity of the Netherlands Nutrition Foundation is the organization of conferences on its own or in combination with other institutions or organizations. An important conference was organized in March 1976 on "The progress towards a food and nutrition policy in The Netherlands". The Foundation took the leadership of this conference and the organization was done in close co-operation with the Netherlands Society for Nutrition and Food Technology.

The Foundation is also involved in the preparation of statements on specific topics which are to be discussed in workshops by a limited number of people. For several months a workshop has been in preparation on the subject of "alcohol and nutrition", to be held in the fall of this year. Several other topics are on our list for the coming years.

We are at present also discussing whether the Foundation should take leadership in an activity that I should like to describe as follows. As you know, at regular times all kind of "nonsense" is written or told about food and nutrition, not only by lay people but also by people with academical qualifications or by industries. In the Netherlands there is no organization which could prepare at very short notice a statement in which the "nonsense" is indicated by using proper scientifically based information. This proper information could be distributed to the known communication channels. We wonder whether this is a task of the Nutrition Foundation and what could be the disadvantages of such an activity.

6. Most Foundations have their own publication organs, like *Nutrition Reviews, British Nutrition Foundation Bulletin, Näringsforskning.*

Our Foundation has no own publication organ, but on the other hand, it has a very good relationship with *The Netherlands Journal of Nutrition (Voeding)* in which we can publish specific information.

I do not think that we should try to publish our own Bulletin in the near future; perhaps we should try, if a kind of formal link with *The Netherlands Journal of Nutrition* is possible.

7. Finally, I should like to mention here the very good contacts we had in the past years with the American, British and Swedish Nutrition Foundations. Our Foundation has been lately in a transitional phase: we have had to work hard on a new future in which we have dared to take the leadership in specific fields of nutrition, keeping in mind that our ultimate goal is improvement of human nutritional health. The good contacts with the other Foundations helped us very much in identifying our future responsibilities. For their help I should like to thank them very much and I hope that we, as an informal group of nutrition foundations, will continue our work together.

Our work in the future should also be done in close contact with other organizations in the field of nutrition. We can even say that the success of our work will depend upon the relationships we have with those other organizations.

8. *Additional information*

Members of the Board (dated September 1977)

Dr. M. G. L. van Schouwenburg, President.
Mr. J. C. van Beek, Treasurer
Professor Dr. J. G. A. J. Hautvast, Secretary General
Professor Dr. G. den Boef
Professor Dr. Ir. M. J. L. Dols
Professor Dr. C. den Hartog
Professor Dr. R. Luyken
Professor Dr. R. Zielhuis
Dr. M. E. J. Hijmans, Advisor
Dr. A. de Wit-Elshove, Secretary

Secretarial address:

Professor Dr. J. G. A. J. Hautvast

Dept. of Human Nutrition of The Agricultural University
De Dreijen II
Wageningen, The Netherlands
Telephone: 08370-82590 (82589)

"Netherlands Nutrition Foundation" Chair, University of Amsterdam:

1947-1972	Professor Dr. Ir. M. J. L. Dols
1972-...	Professor Dr. R. Luyken

The Swedish Nutrition Foundation

Leif Hambraeus

Professor of Human Nutrition, University of Uppsala
Sweden, and Executive Officer of the Swedish Nutrition Foundation,
Uppsala, Sweden

Until 1970 human nutrition was a fairly little favoured branch of science within Sweden. Except for a Food and Vitamin section within the National Institute of Public Health, which mainly had a controlling function, there were no professorships or departments of human nutrition established until July 1970. However, in 1970 three chairs in nutrition were established within the medical faculties at the universities of Gothenburg, Lund and Uppsala, respectively. Each of them were given its own profile. Thus the institute in Gothenburg was devoted to clinical nutrition, the institute in Lund, which is common to the medical and technical faculties, is devoted to industrial nutrition and the one in Uppsala is devoted to nutritional problems of infancy and childhood as well as international nutrition problems with special reference to the developing countries. A fourth chair in nutrition was established a few years later at the Caroline Institute in Stockholm devoted to medical nutrition and public health nutrition problems. Furthermore, a new food legislation was adopted in Sweden in 1972 and a National Food Administration was established to succeed the National Institute of Public Health. The National Food Administration moved into a new building in Uppsala in 1975.

How it Started

Already in 1953 a working group of medical, agricultural and food industry representatives outlined on their own initiative the organization of a national institute of human nutrition, which should be financed partly by the food industries and partly by the Government. The detailed plans were forwarded to the Government in 1955. The plans were widely approved of those concerned but for various reasons the Government did not carry them further, one of the reasons obviously being that a governmental committee had been established for the outline of a proper organization of nutrition research and education within Sweden. In order to keep up the interest and support for nutrition research within Sweden the above-mentioned working group then directed their efforts towards the establishment of a Nutrition Foundation which was modelled in principle on the same basis as its American equivalent, the Nutrition Foundation of the United States, which started in 1941.

As a result of the enthusiastic efforts of one of the food industry leaders, Mr. Lars Anderfelt, the Swedish Nutrition Foundation was established in December 1961 at a meeting in Stockholm where representatives of fourteen food and related industries participated and accepted their responsibility as sponsors for the Foundation. A number of academic scientists with an interest in nutrition as well as representatives of the governmental agencies were also present and Dr. C. G. King, who was at that time President and scientific director of the US Nutrition Foundation, stood as godfather.

Aim

The Foundation was originally intended to promote scientific research within nutrition and nearby fields of interest for the food industry, food producers and other enterprisers who have an interest to follow the development within the field of nutrition research.

The Foundation should furthermore promote the potential use and practical application of scientific results obtained within the field of nutrition. The wording of the statutes and bylaws are to some extent influenced by the taxation regulations within Sweden. This does not, however, prevent a wide diversification of the Foundation's ways and means of supporting nutrition research.

The Foundation was, as has been pointed out earlier, established almost a decade before there were any nutrition institutions founded within the medical faculties at our universities and it has, without any doubt, played a very essential role in the stimulation of nutrition research within our country. Furthermore, it has probably also indirectly helped to open the eyes of our government to the need of nutrition research and education within the universities.

Organization

The original fourteen members or sponsors of the Foundation have now increased to twenty-five. The members represent food companies including food producers, suppliers, distributors and processors. The Foundation has its office in Uppsala.

The objectivity of the opinions and actions of the Foundation is ensured by its board and by its committees where prominent and independent scientists within the field of human nutrition participate.

The Foundation is governed by a Board of Trustees which meets at least once a year. Each economic contributor is allowed to select one member of the Board of Trustees. At their annual meeting the Board of Trustees elect members of the Governing Body. In this half of the members should represent the member companies and the other half scientists from public institutions and universities or representatives of governmental agencies. The Chairman is a public representative, it has so far been the Governor of the County of Uppsala.

The Foundation is actively led by an Executive Officer who should be appointed by the Governing Body. The Executive Officer should be or should have been actively working as a scientist. He has the full responsibility of all the activities of the Foundation between the meetings of the Board of Trustees and the Governing Body, as well as for the current administrative work and for book-keeping and management of the funds.

The Executive Officer is an *ex-officio* member of the Governing Body. The Executive Officer has to help an Executive Committee as well as a Scientific Advisory Committee and a Food Industries Advisory Committee. The Executive Officer is *ex-officio* member of all these committees. The Scientific Advisory Committee comprises eleven scientists active in nutrition research. They meet about four times a year to decide on matters which need consideration and approval from scientific expertise, e.g. research grants and stipends, planning of symposia or other matters which are submitted to them by the governing body.

The Executive Committee comprises nine persons and has to represent the governing body between its meetings. Half of the members are representatives for the economic sponsors, half of them are academic scientists working at the universities. The Chairman is one of the representatives of the food industry.

The Food Industries Advisory Committee comprises twenty-one members, one for each sponsoring industry, and is meant to provide a direct contact between members and technical leaders of the industries and the university nutrition scientists.

Economy

The budget is covered by member fees from Swedish or multinational food industries who market food products in Sweden, as well as from food producers and the farmers' organization. The annual budget for 1977 comprises totally 780,000 Swedish Crowns which is equivalent to about US$160,000 with the addition of 200,000 Swedish Crowns (± US$40,000) for the support of pediatric nutrition research (see below).

The Foundation has the rights to receive contributions for the furthering of its activities, provided that no conditions have been prescribed that the Board considers to be against the purpose of the Foundation. An individual member or sponsor of the Foundation is not allowed to contribute with a current amount exceeding half of the total current contributions if there are no special reasons or/and it has not been accepted by the governing body. The governing body has, however, the liberty to receive further support above that of the Foundation's account for special purposes, i.e. for the activity of affiliated bodies. Contributions to the Foundation can, of course, not be returned.

Adhering Bodies

During the last few years it has been felt that the Swedish Nutrition Foundation could also serve as a mother organization or a coordinator of scientific advisory boards and nutrition foundations which are devoted to specific nutrition problems. This would provide the possibility of exchange of views and knowledge and also to coordinate the grants given to nutrition research from different bodies.

Thus a special Scientific Advisory Board for cereal products was established in 1975 by the Bread Institute in collaboration with SNF. The Bread Institute represents an organization sponsored by the cereal producers and the bakery industry in order to promote bread consumption and to increase the knowledge of cereal products and their use in the Swedish diet.

This advisory board comprises two Professors of Nutrition, one of them being the executive officer of the Swedish Nutrition Foundation, one is Professor of Caryology and one Professor of Plant Breeding. A specific Foundation for pediatric nutrition research was established in 1976 in collaboration with the Swedish Nutrition Foundation and the two baby-food companies in Sweden, Findus and Semper. This Foundation gives research grants and stipends to persons engaged in the nutritional problems of infancy and childhood. The Foundation is partly administered by the office of the Swedish Nutrition Foundation.

Activities

The Swedish Nutrition Foundation is working mainly along three different lines:

1. The publication of a specific bulletin *Näringsforskning (Nutrition Research).*
2. Support of research and travel grants.
3. The arrangement of international and national symposia and conferences.

1. Publication Activities

The bulletin *Näringsforskning (Nutrition Research)* is published 4 times a year. It has an edition comprising 3000 copies including about 1250 subscribers. It is also distributed free of charge to most libraries and hospitals and to several public libraries as well as to some scientific institutions and to schools of home economics. Originally it was almost

100 per cent a reference journal with almost no original articles. However, it has during the last few years changed somewhat and contains today original studies regarding nutritional problems of local interest for Sweden and the Scandinavian countries, in addition to review articles in the field of nutrition. During the last few years summaries to theses presented within the scope of nutrition within Sweden have also been published in the journal. The journal also functions as the mouthpiece of the Swedish Nutrition Association and publishes abstracts of lectures and communications presented at their meetings. The articles are usually written in Scandinavian language but for the last 5 years they have had a summary in English. Occasionally articles are also printed completely in the English language. With the exception of a few years the executive officer also functions as the editor of the journal. Otherwise there is no special editorial staff and consequently there are problems around the practical work and advanced discussions have started to coproduce the journal with another journal run by a related organization for rationalization and efficient editorial assistance.

2. *Support of Research*

Since the establishment of the Foundation a certain amount of money is devoted as support to research work in basic as well as applied nutrition. From the beginning the amount was 150,000 Swedish Crowns (equivalent to US$30,000) and this is distributed in individual grants varying between 4000 Sw.Cr. (US$800) and 12,000 Sw.Cr. (US$2500) annually. The receivers have to present their results in reports for publication in the bulletin and/or in the Swedish Nutrition Foundation annual report. These grants undoubtedly have played a significant role in stimulating nutrition research especially for young scientists. However, during the 15 years that have passed since the Foundation was established the total amount has not increased in absolute terms and this means that inflation has almost ruined even the best intentions of the Foundation to support research. It is therefore under discussion whether this support of basic nutrition research should be revitalized which would necessitate a considerable increase of the member fees of the Foundation or be rearranged.

Travel grants and stipends are bestowed for participation in conferences and congresses or for short visits to laboratories outside Sweden. Young scientists are favoured. During 1975 five grants for the participation in the international Nutrition Congress in Japan were given. For 1977 a total amount of 20,000 Swedish Crowns (4.000 U$) is devoted to travel grants and stipends.

3. Arrangement of Symposia and Conferences

The Swedish Nutrition Foundation has perhaps established its special profile through the arrangement of international symposia on nutritional issues of common interest. The proceedings of the symposia are published as monographs in the series *Symposia of the Swedish Nutrition Foundation.* During 1962-1973 international symposia have been held every year but due to economic restrictions they have only been held every second year since 1973.

The various topics dealt with are listed in Table 1. In 1977 the year's symposium was titled "The Mother and Child Dyad/ Nutritional Aspects". It was held in Uppsala in June in the University Building due to the fact that Uppsala University celebrated its 500th anniversary in 1977. Previously the meetings have been held at various resort places in Sweden. We were extremely happy that the Nutrition Foundation's reprint of Rosén von Rosenstein's *Textbook on Diseases of Children* and their remedies, which was first published in 1776, was made available to the symposium. Rosén von Rosenstein was Professor at the University of Uppsala in medicine.

Table 1

Symposia of the Swedish Nutrition Foundation

Year	Title
1961	Mild-Moderate Forms of Protein-Calorie Malnutrition
1962	Occurrence, Causes and Prevention of Overnutrition
1963	Nutrition and Caries Prevention
1964	Polyunsaturated Fatty Acids as Nutrients
1965	Nutrition and Physical Activity

Table 1 (cont.)

1966	Occurrence, Causes and Prevention of Nutritional Anemias
1967	Nutrition in Preschool and School Age
1968	Food Cultism and Nutrition Quackery
1969	Famine. A Symposium dealing with Nutrition and Relief Operations in Times of Disaster
1970	Nutrition in Old Age
1971	Intestinal Enzyme Deficiencies and their Nutritional Implications
1973	Early Malnutrition and Mental Development
1975	Food and Immunology
1977	The Mother/Child Dyad—Nutritional Implications

It has, however, been discussed that it would be advantageous if the Swedish Nutrition Foundation also dealt more actively with national nutrition problems and questions. We have therefore since 1973 also arranged more nationally oriented conferences, usually held in Stockholm, the capital of Sweden. Most of them have been arranged in collaboration with the National Board of Health and Welfare. The proceedings have then been published in the journal *Näringsforskning*. The topics of the seminars so far held are shown in Table 2. This autumn we are planning a seminar on the "Nutrition policy and food consumption in Sweden". This certainly has an international aspect but in this seminar we will especially discuss how far we have gone in Sweden with respect to the establishment of a food and nutrition policy and what we now know about the effect of food subsidies.

Table 2

Nationally oriented symposia arranged by the Swedish Nutrition Foundation

1974	Prevention of Iron Deficiency in Sweden by means of a Better Diet
1975	Nutrition Education in the Faculties of Medicine in Sweden
1976	Nutrition and Food Marketing
1977	Nutrition Policy and Food Consumption in Sweden

Administration

As Sweden is a small country the Swedish Nutrition Foundation obviously has a much smaller dimension than its American opposite and the Swedish Nutrition Foundation has always had a very small organization. The personnel comprises one person with an academic background and university status, i.e. the executive officer, as well as a secretary. The first executive officer of the Foundation was Professor Gunnar Blix, one of the founders of SNF who worked part time after his retirement from his chair in medical biochemistry at the University of Uppsala. He was succeeded in 1971 by Professor Lars A. Carlsson, who was Professor of Geriatrics at the University of Uppsala. At that time the responsibility as the editor of the journal was separated and taken over by myself. Since 1973 I have myself been the executive officer and editor of the journal besides my ordinary work as Professor of Human Nutrition at the University of Uppsala. At the secretariat we have only one person appointed, Mrs Sylvia Molin, who was earlier on part time but today full time. In addition we have a part-time assistant paid by the Social Services of the Government.

It is quite obvious that the small personnel hampers our activities and best intentions and the increasing cost of labour, in addition to the heavily increasing printing costs, secondary to inflation, has led to a situation where the whole organization of the activities of the Foundation has to be carefully re-evaluated.

At the yearly meeting of the Trustees in April 1977 it was therefore decided that a special working committee should look over the Foundation and present a plan of reorganization. For taxation reasons the purpose of the Foundation could not be changed more than to a certain degree. It would be honest to say that it has even been discussed whether the Foundation should cease, but I am happy to say that it was unanimously felt that the Foundation still wanted to survive and that the trustees were more interested to revitalize it than to kill it off. It is obvious from discussions with the trustees that they are most interested in keeping the journal published as well as keeping the seminar activities going.

It is obvious that most of the trustees, as well as the members of the governing body, felt that the role of the Swedish Nutrition Foundation as a transmitter of nutrition information, independent of both commerce and government, has great value for all those who seek an unbiased view on nutritional matters. It was therefore felt that it would be desirable if in the future the SNF should endeavour to expand its activities in the field of nutrition information both towards professional and laymen. Consequently it was felt essential that the editorial problems of *Näringsforskning* were solved firstly, and secondly, that the nationally oriented seminar activities were expanded if necessary at the cost of the grants for nutrition research which today seem to have lost their initiator role.

With respect to the grants and stipends, however, it is being discussed whether some other type of purpose should be tried. It should be remembered that when the Foundation was instituted there were no institutes of nutrition established within the country. Today there are four and thus it might be more meaningful to stimulate other activities to help the institutes than just giving out minor grants which, due to inflation, mean very little today.

The Swiss Nutrition Foundation and the General Role of Foundations in Supporting Biomedical Research

Hugo E. Aebi

Professor of Biochemistry, Berne University, Switzerland, President of the Swiss Science Council, President of the Swiss Nutrition Foundation

In this contribution three points are discussed which are of relevance for any institution supporting research. First, the creation of the Swiss Nutrition Foundation, serving as an example of what can be done whenever a certain discipline is underdeveloped or underrated. Second, the role of nutrition in biomedical research as well as in the medical curriculum. Third, the problem of setting priorities in science policy in general and in nutrition research in particular.

I. The Swiss Nutrition Foundation

The fact that Switzerland is a confederation with rather decentralized political power is also reflected in science inasmuch as several organisms exist, competences and tasks being more or less clearly divided between them. The creation of the Swiss Nutrition Foundation in 1968 may be regarded as the result of a joint venture. Before 1968 there were three organizations involved in nutrition, though in different ways: (1) The Federal Commission of Nutrition (Eidg. Ernährungskommission), created in 1949 by decision of the Federal Government, is a consulting board whose main task it is to advise the Federal Office of Public Health in all matters of nutrition and food legislation. (2) The Swiss Society for Nutrition Research, founded in 1953 by the initiative of Fritz Verzàr, Professor of Physiology at Basel University, is a scientific society in the strict sense of the word. (3) The Swiss Association for Nutrition (Schweiz. Vereinigung für Ernährung), founded in 1965, has as its main aim the propagation and dissemination of knowledge related to nutrition and health in general. Representatives of all three organizations met on March 18, 1967 in order to examine the general situation in nutrition research, which was considered to be unsatisfactory. Scientists felt unhappy because of the insufficient infrastructure available for nutrition research at the universities and because of almost complete lack of systematic teaching of nutrition and food sciences at the universities. In contrast to the flourishing and powerful enterprises of the pharmaceutical and food industries there was hardly any counterpart in the institutions of higher teaching. Since no special funds were available for research projects in nutrition, it was felt that a joint venture was badly needed. A working group who had the task to study possible steps to be taken came to the conclusion that a centralized solution, i.e. the creation of a national center, was out of the question. However, the plan of establishing a Foundation was considered to be compatible with Switzerland's federalistic structure and therefore met everybody's approval. Thanks to good relations between the main representatives in industrial companies and at the universities the necessary funds could be raised and appropriate by-laws were prepared (Fig. 1).

The council of the Foundation met for the first time on February 20, 1969; on the same day legal steps were taken to officially establish the Swiss Nutrition Foundation (Verurkundung durch Notar). A few weeks later the Foundation was presented to the public; the first speaker at this meeting being a member of the Federal Government, Bundesrat Tschudi, Minister of Education and Science at that time. In his inauguration speech he pointed out that promoting scientific research is a common task of both government and private industry and that partnership between economy and science is a good thing, provided that they help and respect each other. In his considerations he also concluded that this co-operation can best be accomplished in the form of a private Foundation. The legal basis of the Swiss Nutrition Foundation is two-fold: the by-laws of the Foundation on the one hand and the

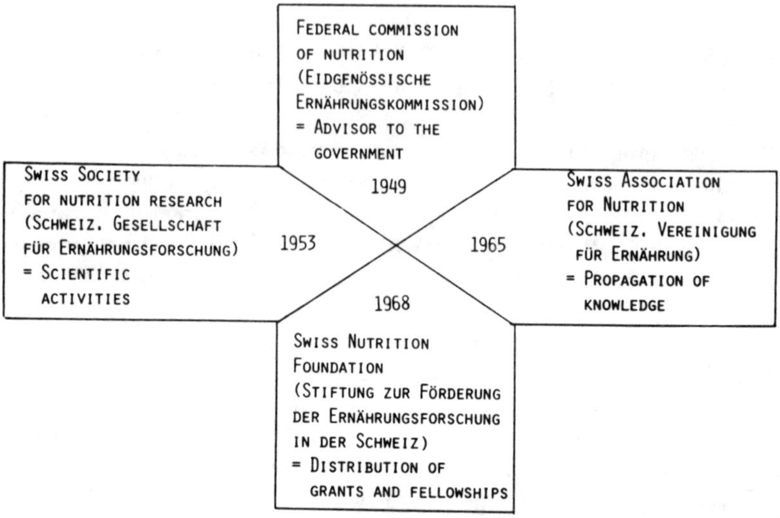

Fig. 1. Research in nutrition and food sciences in Switzerland: distribution of tasks.

general conditions imposed by the federal authorities on private Foundations of any kind on the other. The by-laws are simple and flexible, so that rapid and efficient help can be given to the scientists. Article 2 of the by-laws runs as follows: "The Swiss Nutrition Foundation has the purpose to promote research in the entire field of nutrition. In particular this is done by (1) providing qualified applicants with grants for experimental or clinical research as well as for field studies which are likely to give new insights. (2) Scholarships are offered young university graduates in order to recruit well-qualified and motivated candidates for special training in nutrition. (3) Publication grants may be awarded in order to propagate relevant results obtained in nutrition research."

It is the policy of the Foundation that the main emphasis of its activity be put on the scholarship programme. In this context young university graduates were invited to attend the annual post-graduate course in nutrition at the University of Cambridge. This possibility of receiving special training in the field of nutrition is used increasingly. At first, no candidates were interested in such a scholarship; however, since 1972 the number of applicants has always exceeded the two fellowships available every year. So far ten fellows have successfully attended this course and obtained the diploma. Most of them obtained adequate positions either in industry or university institutions. Unfortunately, the continuation of this policy is being questioned and possible alternatives are being examined at present.

The Foundation's budget is based on an annual income of Sw. Fr. 158,000.-. One part of this sum consists of the interests of the Foundation's capital (Fr. 500,000) and the other part is raised by annual contributions. From a financial point of view, too, this Foundation is the achievement of a common effort. There are seven companies of the Swiss food industry who have provided the Foundation's capital and continue to contribute annually: Nestlé-Alimentana and Hoffmann-La Roche (category I), Wander, Haco, Knorr, Sais-Astra, Suchard-Tobler (category II). At present the former contribute 37,500.- francs and the latter 12,500.- francs per year. This uneven figure is due to the fact that 2 years ago the donors unanimously agreed to increase their donations by 25 per cent. Since the expenses for administration can be kept to an absolute minimum about 150,000 francs are available every year for research projects and fellowships.

In the 8 years of its existence the Foundation has contributed the sum of 1 million francs for the realization of about twenty research projects, besides the ten fellowships awarded. This is a relatively modest sum, if compared to the amount spent by other institutions supporting research. Nevertheless, in quite a few instances it successfully acted as a trigger, which is, in fact, the real goal of this institution.

II. The Role of Nutrition in Biomedical Research and in the Medical Curriculum

Assuming that, even today, in a university teaching and research have to go together, there must be close links between these two main activities in academic life. Stimulating teaching favours the motivation of good students and therefore provides new collaborators. Consequently there are two good reasons to include teaching nutrition in the medical curriculum:

1. Nutrition must be considered as the most important environmental factor forming and influencing the human organism.

2. The standard of nutrition research ultimately depends on the number and skill of young physicians and scientists determined to do research work in nutrition.

In the medical curriculum the teaching of basic facts of nutrition can be done at the preclinical, the clinical and the post-graduate level. Since the author is teaching at the preclinical level this phase of the medical curriculum shall serve as an example. At Berne University nutrition and digestion are taught in the second year in a separate block. This consists of a series of lectures following the system of integrated teaching. Whereas digestion is mainly taught by the anatomist and the physiologist, nutrition is mainly given by the biochemist. There are several good opportunities to combine metabolic and nutritional aspects; e.g. the dynamic state of body constituents. The way how it may serve as a unifying link is shown in Fig. 2. Besides these lectures the students have to perform analyses of some important foods (e.g. potato, milk, meat, vegetables) in the practical class. For the written examination in biochemistry the multiple-choice procedure is used, 20 out of 100 questions being related to nutrition. In the practical examination at the end of the second year the student may have to carry out food analyses.

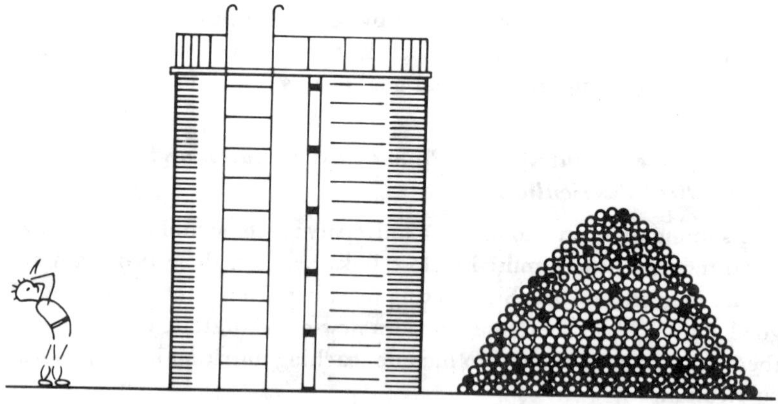

Fig. 2. Body constituents and food intake in a period of 65 years (=24,000d).

Nutrition teaching in the preclinical part of the medical curriculum should comprise the following items:

1. Basic facts about food and nutrition:

   - Knowledge of the nutritive value and the essential composition of main food stuffs (e.g. cereals, milk, meat, fruit, vegetable).
   - Composition and design of a normal balanced diet and how to get this message to the layman.
   - Knowledge of the need for single dietary components and their limits and risks.

2. Digestion and metabolic regulation: Unless taught at the clinical level this part should also include the role of the composition of the meal and the effect of the food-intake schedule on metabolism.

3. Additives and residues.
   This should also include possible hazards of such substances. The essentials regarding food legislation must be taught too.

4. Psychological and social aspects. It is felt that this is an important complementary aspect to biochemical and metabolic facts on nutrition.

5. Malnutrition. Unless there are special reasons for teaching this item at the clinical level, the section on protein metabolism and on energy balance should be complemented by lectures on the consequences of undernutrition (PCM) and overnutrition (e.g. obesity). The latter can preferentially be accomplished jointly with representatives of clinical disciplines.

6. Diet prophylaxis of metabolic diseases, in particular of enzyme-deficiency conditions, can easily be fitted into the lectures on enzymes or on genetic problems. These topics represent an excellent opportunity to establish a close link between basic biochemical knowledge and medical practice and public health (e.g. PKU).

What is the general situation regarding teaching nutrition in medical schools today? In order to answer this question the outcome of two meetings may be quoted where this has been discussed in some detail. On May 5 and 6 a group of about 200 nutrition experts met in Geneva at the thirtieth assembly of the World Health Organization. Divided into eight groups they analysed the present situation. Among many other things it was stated that not enough attention is paid to nutrition in medical education at all levels. This crucial question was discussed in some more detail by a small working group on behalf of the international union of nutritional sciences. This workshop was mainly intended to locate the gaps and shortcomings and to propose possible ways how to overcome them. There was an unanimous opinion that in most curricula nutrition is represented in an insufficient manner. Therefore it was felt that additional efforts are mandatory to correct this lack of information. The chairman of this meeting, Professor Cremer of the University of Giessen, has prepared a report which is being submitted to the President of the WHO expert group (Professor Gopalan, India, President of IUNS). In this context a statement made by an African colleague was most impressing. He stated that nutrition is an under-rated science, not only in the curriculum of many European universities, but also in those of the medical schools in developing countries.

Obviously it would be unrealistic, or even utopic, to wait for the result of such recommendations. Therefore the author would like to make a plea to all those colleagues who are responsible for the elaboration or reformation of medical curricula. What can be done at the faculty level, especially by means of a policy of small steps, should be accomplished without delay. There are a good deal of appropriate opportunities at the preclinical as well as at the clinical level. Especially at this later stage of medical education, teaching related to food intake should not be restricted to dietetics as part of therapy, but should include nutrition at large, this being an important part of primary health care. The notion that good nutrition is one of the main prerequisites for man's health should have as a consequence that nutrition, a basic as well as mission-oriented science, has an appropriate place in the curriculum of the young physician.

III. The Activity of Private Foundations; Their Role in a National Science Policy

For any highly industrialized country adequate support of research is a task of crucial importance. Usually this is done jointly by the government and its organizations as well as by the private industry. Switzerland represents a special case inasmuch as the total expenses for research and development are mainly met by the private sector (industry, economy, etc., *ca.* 80 per cent): the confederation and the cantons contribute only 20 per cent of this sum. The total costs for research and development are estimated to be 3.5 billion Sw. francs, which corresponds to about 2½ per cent of the gross national product. The main task of any national science policy is not only to mobilize all sources for supporting research, but even more so to assure that the funds, whether public or private, are efficiently used. This in turn requests a careful selection of research proposals together with a reasonable system of setting priorities. All those measures to be taken within the system of a national research policy should be aimed at securing an adequate research potential in our country at a reasonable cost. This research potential has a twofold task: (1) participation in and contribution to the worldwide scientific progress; (2) production of scientific results relevant to the solution of the problems of our society (Fig. 3).

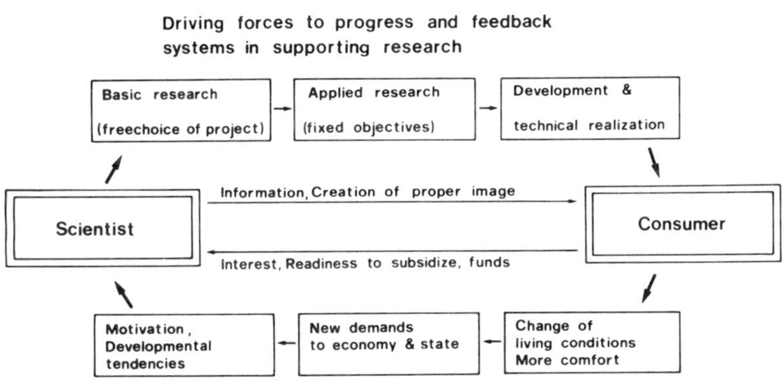

Fig. 3. Driving forces to progress and feedback systems in supporting research.

The particular situation in nutrition research reflects this general picture to some extent. Extensive research in nutrition and food sciences is performed in the laboratories of the big companies of the food industry as well as the pharmaceutical enterprises. In companies like Nestlé and Hoffmann-La Roche there are excellent research groups who are working in the front line of progress. This is particularly true for the development of milk products, convenience food, beverages, production of vitamins and low-calorie food. Additional efforts to promote nutrition research have been made by the private industry in two ways: the creation of a number of Foundations supporting biomedical research at large and one supporting nutrition research in particular. In this context the creation of the Institute for Nutrition Research by the Green Meadow Foundation in Rüschlikon Zürich has to be mentioned too.

The setting of priorities in research is a tedious and difficult task since clear-cut decisions are often hampered by political or individual constraints. If it is accepted that all research projects aimed at improving the living conditions of man should get a high degree of priority this is particularly true for nutrition, food science and all the related topics. How is the setting of priorities done in Swiss science policy? Decisions have to be made at three levels: (1) The decision how much of the total public funds should be spent for research and development at large is a strictly political issue. In Switzerland this decision is taken by the Parliament when the annual budget is approved and when special issues are discussed. (2) The distribution of the available funds among the different sectors and disciplines requires a decision to be taken jointly by politicians and scientists. In basic research this is done by the National Research Council who has to submit its annual distribution plan to the Federal authorities. This plan consists of a carefully equilibrated budget indicating how much money will be available for research projects in groups of disciplines, such as chemistry, physics or biology. Before the final decision is taken the Swiss Science Council will be consulted. (3) The allocation of funds within a discipline is a delicate but important matter, which should remain entirely in the hands of scientists. This is true, for example, for the evaluation of projects submitted to the Swiss National Science Foundation. The only criterium that should be considered at this level is quality. This includes the competence of the scientist, the originality of the research project and perhaps the feasibility of the proposed study related to the available facilities (Fig. 4).

Since the proper selection of projects and a fair distribution of the available funds is the main domain of any private Foundation, the above considerations are also of crucial importance for any nutrition Foundation. The difficulty that may arise in supporting nutrition research is just what makes nutrition so interesting a topic in teaching

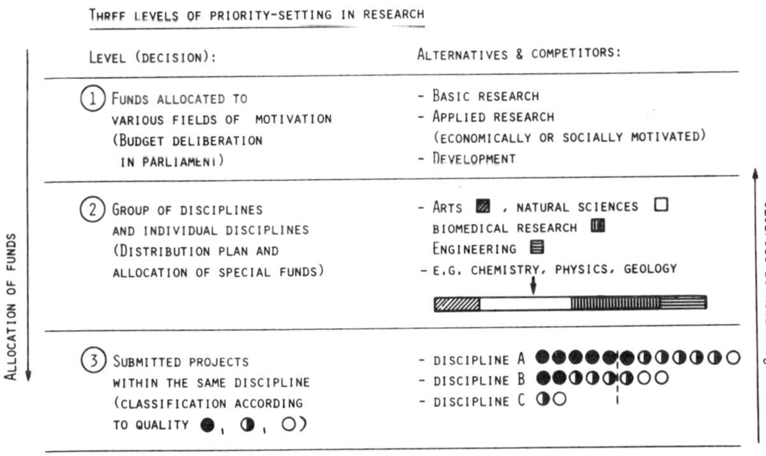

Fig. 4. Three levels of priority-setting in research

and research. It is an interdisciplinary science by definition covering a large area, from basic science, such as biochemistry and physiology, to clinical as well as social and preventive medicine. So there are quite a number of disciplines which may eventually claim to get additional support from a nutrition Foundation. Consequently, the most important but also the most delicate task will be the proper selection of the projects or other activities to be subsidized. Considering that the main message in teaching nutrition is the plea for a well-balanced diet, this sound rule should also be followed when limited funds are distributed. The aim shall be not to scatter indefinitely the limited means, but rather select the most promising projects and give them a chance. It is in this sense that the Swiss sister Foundation wishes a good start. May the work of the Nutrition Foundation of Italy be successful and most beneficial to the scientific community active in nutrition research in this country.

Bibliography

1. *Stiftung zur Förderung der Ernährungsforschung in der Schweiz; Berichterstattung über die Tätigkeit 1969-1974.* Address: Medizinisch-chemisches Institut, Postfach 3000 Bern 9.

2. *Schriftenreihe der schweizerischen Vereinigung für Ernährung,*

Hefte 1-37. Address: Eidg. Alkoholverwaltung, Postfach 3000 Bern 9.

3. *Forschungsbericht des Schweiz. Wissenschaftsrates,* Bern, 1973. Address: Schweiz. Wissenschaftsrat, Postfach 2732, 3001 Bern.

4. *Jahresbericht 1976, Schweiz. Nationalfonds zur Förderung der wissenschaftlichen Forschung.* Address: Wildhainweg 20, 3001 Bern.

5. *Zur Ernährungssituation der schweizerischen Bevölkerung (erster schweizerischer Ernährungsbericht)* (eds. G. Brubacher and G. Ritzel), Verlag Hans Huber, Bern, 1975.

6. *Ernährung und Gesundheitszustand der Bergbevölkerung der Schweiz* (eds. F. Verzar and D. Gsell), Verlag der Eidg. Drucksachen- und Material-Zentrale, Bern, 1962.

7. *Food and Nutrition Research,* Report of the ARC/MRC Committee, Elsevier Scientific Publishing Company, Amsterdam, New York, 1974.

8. *Medical Research Systems in Europe,* Ciba Foundation Symposium 21 (new series), Elsevier, Excerpta Medica, North Holland, Amsterdam, London, New York, 1973.

9. *Guide to European Foundations,* prepared by the Giovanni Agnelli Foundation (ed. Franco Angeli), Milano, 1973.

10. *Science in Switzerland,* by J. M. Luck, Columbia University Press, 1967.

11. Background document for reference and use at the technical discussions on "the importance of national and international food and nutrition policies for health development"; WHO; A30/Technical Discussions/1, 21 March 1977.

Nutrition Research in Spain

Francisco Grande

Instituto de Bioquímica y Nutrición, Fundación F. Cuenca Villoro, and Department of Biochemistry, Faculty of Sciences, University of Zaragoza, Zaragoza, 6. Spain

I should like to thank Professor Rodolfo Paoletti, and the Nutrition Foundation of Italy, for inviting me to be here today. It is indeed a pleasure to be present at this meeting and I have enjoyed very much the presentations of those who have preceded me.

Regretfully, I have to take in my presentation a different approach than that taken by the previous speakers. I cannot speak of the Spanish Nutrition Foundation, for the simple reason that such a Foundation does not exist. There is no public or private organization in Spain for promoting teaching and research in nutrition; and it should be recognized that the Spanish contribution to nutrition has been rather modest and discontinuous.

Under these circumstances, I shall devote the time assigned to me reviewing some historical highlights of nutritional research in Spain and making a few comments about the present situation on nutritional teaching and research in that country.

Historically, Spain's main contribution to human nutrition is related to her role in the introduction to Europe of some New World foods which, eventually, became an important part of the European diet. Among them potatoes and corn deserve special consideration.

Potatoes were grown in Spain shortly after Columbus' first trips. By 1573 potatoes were an important part of the diet of the Hospital de la Sangre in Seville. There is no need to tell you about the important role of potatoes, as a source of calories and vitamin C, in the diet of the Central and Northern European countries, and all of you are, no doubt, familiar with the story of the Irish potato famine (1845), which shows the importance of the potato crop for the nutrition of the Irish people.

The introduction of corn is, perhaps, of more interest from the viewpoint of nutritional research, in connection with the problem of pellagra. By the eighteenth century corn was cultivated extensively in northern Spain and northern Italy. Italy and Spain, indeed, share the common fate of being the two countries where this disease was first observed and studied. It may be appropriate to remind you of some of the highlights of the history of pellagra.

The History of Pellagra *in Spain*

The first clinical description of pellagra, as all of you know, was made by Gaspar Casal, a Spanish physician working in Oviedo, the capital of the province of Asturias in northern Spain which happens to be the province where I was born. The original description was made in 1735, but it was not published until 1762, 3 years after Casal's death in Madrid. This description of Pellagra appears in a book entitled *Historia Natural y Médica del Principado de Asturias* ("Natural and Medical History of the Principality of Asturias", Madrid, 1762). In the original description, written in Latin, Casal used the popular name given by the Asturian peasants to the disease, that is "Mal de la Rosa", or "rose's disease", a name that alludes to the pink colour of the early cutaneous symptoms of the disease. The name pellagra was introduced by the Italian physician Francesco Frapolli in 1771 and is, of course, the name universally used ever since.

It is interesting to note the great variety of popular names given to the disease in different parts of Italy and Spain, and the correspondence of these names between the two countries. Thus, the Italian name "salso", which alludes to the salty taste, corresponds to the Spanish name of "Flema salada" used in the Province of Cuenca. The Italian name "Mal de fegato", or liver disease, corresponds to the Spanish "Mal del hígado", used mainly in Aragón. The name "Mal della testa" (head's disease) corresponds to "Mal de la cabeza", etc.

Due to the great prevalence of pellagra in some areas of the Italian peninsula, there were the Italian physicians who since the end of the eighteenth century and throughout the nineteenth century have made the most important contributions to the study of the disease. It is not my intention to describe now the history of pellagra research in Italy, which I am sure is well known to all of you. It may be of interest, however, to quote from the introduction of the work on *Pellagra* by Doctor G. Antonioni, from Pavia (published here in Milano in 1902), since it gives some idea of the magnitude of the problem at the beginning of the present century:

> "When the month of May flourishes, when the first warm and sunny days bring the hope of the new crops in the plains of Lombardy, stimulating the peasants to work on the land, when life awakens for everybody with the hopes of good returns, and the farmers patiently engage in their labours full of sweat; in the middle of the feast of colour and light, when our wonderful and great Paduan valley looks like a smiling garden in the most beautiful and merry season of the year, a sad and devastating disease spreads death in the middle of so much rejoicing and strength. A terrible disease creeps in the blood of those who with full right expected to enjoy that hour; a menacing ghost rises there: the Pellagra."

These words do not need any comment. They clearly show what pellagra meant for the health of the Italian peasants at the beginning of the century and are, at the same time, a tribute to the poetic inspiration of Doctor Antonioni.

Returning to Spain, it appears that Pellagra was a problem limited to a few provinces and the incidence of pellagra, so far as I know, did not reach the proportions it had in Italy. There were, however, a number of Spanish physicians who throughout the nineteenth century contributed to the clinical study of the disease. Among them I shall recall I. Martínez, H. Campo and J. R. Villargoitia in Asturias, Eximeno and Calmarza in Aragón, Olavide and Méndez, Alvaro in Castille, etc. Most of the work of these physicians was related to the clinical description of the disease and the discussion of its identity with the Italian pellagra, but it did not contribute to the knowledge of the pathogenesis of the disease. The most distinguished of these physicians was F. Roel, who in 1880 published in Oviedo a large volume with the title *Etiología de la Pellagra o sea de la pluralidad de enfermedades que aflijen al linaje humano* ("Etiology of Pellagra, or the plurality of diseases which afflict mankind"). I received some information about Roel through my maternal grandfather, who was also a physician as well as the Chairman of the provincial government of Asturias. As such, he had under his authority the charity hospitals of the province and knew Roel, who was working in the provincial welfare hospital of Oviedo, the capital of Asturias.

Roel's work is mainly devoted to the differential diagnosis of pellagra and other diseases, particularly leprosy and scurvy. It is of historical interest to remember that the French authors described pellagra with the name of "Lepra Asturiensis" (or Asturian leprosy) and that some of the early Italian authors used the name "Scorbuto alpino" (that is Scurvy of the Alps).

The Spanish work on pellagra became known in Europe mainly through the French physicians. Casal's original observations were reported in France by Thierry, then physician to the French Ambassador to Madrid, where he met Casal, in the Recueil d'observations de medicine de chirurgie et de pharmacie of Paris (January, 1755), 7 years before the publication of Casal's book. Another French physician, Teophyle Roussel, visited Spain in the first part of the nineteenth century publishing a book, *La Pellagre* (Paris, 1845), in which he affirms that the disease described by Casal as "Mal de la Rosa" is identical to the pellagra of the Italian authors. Casal did relate the development of pellagra to the diet and the consumption of corn. However, because the prevalence of the disease was limited to some areas and was not present in others with similar food consumption, he believed also in the influence of the "atmosphere". On the other hand, it is clear that he believed in the curative effect of the diet, as demonstrated by the descriptions of the clinical cases reported in his book.

There is no need to remind you that the identification of pellagra as a deficiency disease was not achieved until 1914-1918, by the pioneering work of Joseph Goldberger.

Except for the work on pellagra and some work on endemic goiter in the 1920s, not much work was done in Spain on human nutrition until the Civil War (1936-1939). As you may recall, Madrid was practically surrounded by Franco's troups from November 1936 until the end of the war, and the civilian population of the city suffered from a number of nutritional diseases. It was my good luck to have had the opportunity of studying these nutritional disturbances, and I should like to give you now a brief account of this work.

Nutritional Diseases during the Spanish Civil War in Madrid

Some time around the spring of 1937 the Republican Government asked Dr. J. Puche, then Professor of Physiology at the University of Valencia, to organize an Institute of Nutrition in order to study the nutritional problems affecting the civilian population. I was then appointed Head of the Physiology Department and Deputy Director of the Institute, in charge of its Madrid branch. With the help of several colleagues, among them the internists F. Jiménez and J. Márquez and the neurologist M. Peraita, we were able to study over 3000 cases of nutritional diseases. We undertook also some prophylactic measures organizing the distribution of cod liver oil and various vitamin preparations among school children, and to the pregnant and lactating mothers attending the centres of maternal health in the city.

The amount of food distributed to the civilian population of Madrid kept decreasing throughout the duration of the war. My calculations indicate that the daily food supply went down from 1514 kcal (about 6 MJ) *per capita* in August of 1937 to 852 kcal (3.6 MJ) in February 1939. The lowest point was observed in December 1938 when it was only 770 kcal (3.2 MJ).

Deficiency diseases appeared in Madrid as two main waves. The first reached its peak in the spring and early summer of 1938 and was made up of cases of classical Pellagra, as well as of a number of clinical pictures related to Pellagra, but lacking the cutaneous manifestations of this disease and characterized by the preponderancy of neurological disorders. The second wave appeared towards the end of 1938 and lasted until the end of the war in April of 1939. Very few manifestations of specific vitamin deficiencies were observed at this time in spite of the continuous decrease of the food supply. The main clinical picture observed during this second period was famine oedema. No beriberi was seen and only a single case of scurvy was detected.

By the end of 1937 I was aware of the identification of nicotinamide as the pellagra-preventing factor by Elvehjem *et al.*, consequently, when the first cases of pellagra appeared in Madrid, I started preparing nicotinic acid. In order to do that I collected all the nicotine I could from the stores of agricultural supplies in Madrid and Valencia and transformed it into nicotinic acid by the nitric acid oxidation method.

We were able to treat a large number of patients and it soon became apparent that nicotinic acid was very effective in the treatment of the classic signs of pellagra (dermatitis, diarrhoea, dementia). The effect of nicotinic acid was particularly dramatic on the mental manifestations of pellagra. Unconscious patients regained consciousness, often after a single injection. Nicotinic acid, however, had no effect on the neurological manifestations seen in association with the classic signs of Pellagra, as well as in cases of the so-called pellagra sine pellagra, with neurological symptomatology.

We became particularly interested in these neurological disturbances which were carefully analyzed by my colleague the neurologist M. Peraita. Neither clinically nor biochemically could they be identified with beriberi. The patients did not benefit by the treatment with vitamin B_1, but showed some improvement with autoclaved yeast. We used the name paresthetic-causalgic syndrome to describe this clinical picture. It was the most common of all the nutritional disturbances studied, as shown in Table 1.

Table 1

Relative incidence of nutritional-deficiency syndromes in 3116 patients in Madrid (Grande and Peraita)

	No. of cases	Per cent
Paraesthetic-causalgic syndrome	713	22.8
Pellagra and "Pellagra sine pellagra"	677	21.7
Retrobulbar neuritis	509	16.3
Famine oedema	461	14.7
Simple glossitis	336	10.7
Haemorrhagic syndrome	71	2.2
Acoustic neuritis	33	1.5
Various deficiencies	316	10.1

It seems clear now that this syndrome is very similar to the so-called "Burning-feet syndrome" observed by various British and Dutch physicians among the Europeans interned in the Japanese concentration camps.

As I have said, our observations indicate that these manifestations are not due to deficiency of vitamin B_1, B_2 or nicotinic acid and that they are alleviated by autoclaved yeast. Some years ago Gopalan had suggested that a similar syndrome could be due to pantothenic acid deficiency.

An excellent analysis of the nutritional neuropathies in wartime with ample reference to our work can be found in the book *Nutritional Disorders of the Nervous System* by J. D. Spillane (Edinburgh, Livingstone, 1947), and in the monograph by H. Smitskamp, A Neurovascular Syndrome Related to Vitamin Deficiency (Amsterdam, Sheltema and Holkema, 1947). On page 52 of the Smitskamp monograph can be read:

> Until recently the burning feet and ocular disturbances were only seen in coloured people living under poor conditions.
>
> The first occurrence of the disease in Europeans was described by Peraita and Grande and Jimenez during the Spanish civil war in Madrid. They noted the association of glossitis and angular stomatitis with loss of visual and auditory acuity, paresthesia, a burning pain in the soles of the feet and ataxia.

Our work on the nutritional neuropathies has been summarized in the book *Vitaminas y sistema nervioso* ("Vitamins and the nervous system") by F. Grande and M. Peraita (Barcelona, Miguel Servet, 1941).

Nutritional Research in Spain after the Civil War

The limitations of food supply during the years that followed the Civil War and our observations in Madrid during the war stimulated some interest in nutritional research, particularly in connection with the problems of rehabilitation of the undernourished. Professor Jiménez Díaz, then Professor of Internal Medicine at Madrid Medical School, and his associated Doctors Ortiz de Landázuri, Lorente, Vivanco and others, made some interesting clinical observations in this respect. The reports of these workers give an excellent account of the problems met when refeeding extremely undernourished subjects, such as prisoners.

The most important contribution of this period was the study of Lathyrism, the spastic paralysis associated with the consumption of *Lathyrus sativus*. In 1941 there was an important outbreak of this disease in the provinces of Toledo and Ciudad Real, south of Madrid. The clinical syndrome was carefully studied and some measures were taken to avoid the consumption of lathyrus peas, which eventually brought the outbreak under control. This prompted some experimental work by Drs. Vivanco and Jiménez Díaz that led to the identification of other disturbances produced by feeding leguminous seeds to rats, such as the so-called "cicerism", produced by chick-peas (*Cicer arietinum*) and to the differentiation between human lathyrism and the experimental lathyrism of the rat produced by feeding sweet peas (*Lathyrus odoratus*). The Spanish authors proposed the name "odoratism" for the latter syndrome, which is very different from human lathyrism.

At the same period I received some financial support from the Rockefeller Foundation and Dr. W. D. Robinson came from the United States to work with me. We carried out some nutritional surveys on the poor districts of Madrid and I became interested in studying the differences in growth between children of different economic levels, which I continued for a couple of years after Dr. Robinson left Spain when the United States entered the war. My work during these years, in collaboration with Dr. J. Rof, dealt mainly with the capillary invasion of the cornea, which proved to be a non-specific sign of malnutrition, and with the incidence of muscle cramps among children on low calcium intakes. We were able to show remarkable differences in weight, height, and osseous development, between school children of different socio-economic levels.

The Last Twenty Years

Only a limited amount of research on nutrition has been conducted in Spain during the last 20 years. It appears that the improvement of the country's food supply has decreased the interest of Spanish physicians in human nutrition.

The most important work during this period was done by Professor G. Varela and his associates at the Department of Animal Physiology of the

School of Pharmacy, University of Granada. Professor Varela is respon sible for the most comprehensive survey of food consumption done in Spain. His data give a good picture of the average food consumption in the various areas of the country some 10 years ago. In addition, Professor Varela and his group have conducted experimental work on several aspects of nutrition including protein nutrition, calcium metabolism and the effect of cooking and processing on the nutritional properties and the acceptability of various foodstuffs. This work is being continued currently at the Department of Animal Physiology of the School of Pharmacy of Madrid University.

I know of no attempt to evaluate the nutritional status of the Spanish population as a whole. In my opinion this information is urgently needed. Some information in this respect has been provided by Doctor Vivanco and his associate Dr. Palacios who, a few years ago, have done various surveys about the nutritional status of school children in Madrid.

The Present Situation

The main reason for the lack of interest of the Spanish physicians in human nutrition seems to be the absence of organized teaching of nutrition in the Spanish medical schools. There is no chair of nutrition in any of the schools at the present time. All the information on nutrition received by the students is disjointly given as a part of the courses on Physiology, Biochemistry, Clinical Medicine and Pediatrics. I consider this as a very serious problem and, since my return to Spain 2 years ago, I have been trying to organize the teaching of human nutrition at the Medical School in Zaragoza, in the hope of setting an example to be followed by other schools. So far I have failed in this endeavour, but I expect to be offering a course on Human Nutrition starting January 1978. This course, for the time being, will be offered as an elective subject at the third-cycle level, that is to medical students who have completed their curriculum and are working towards a doctor's degree. The course will be open to students of Veterinary Medicine and Chemistry at the doctoral level.

By contrast, the teaching of animal nutrition has greatly improved in the Spanish Schools of Veterinary Medicine, which have also instituted departments of Food Biochemistry and Technology. As happens also in other countries, it may be said that Spanish veterinarians know more about animal nutrition than Spanish physicians know about human nutrition.

Another reason for the stagnation of nutrition research in Spain is the lack of interest of the Public Health authorities. A new Institute of Nutrition has been erected by the Public Health Service (Dirección General de Sanidad) near Madrid. I am not familiar with the work done there, but it seems that the main activity of the centre is concerned with problems of food sanitation and the analytical control of dietetic preparations. As far as I know no experimental work on nutrition is performed there and, to my knowledge, no attempt has been made by the Public Health Service to study the nutritional situation of the Spanish population.

An encouraging sign is the interest shown by a few internists working on the epidemiology and cardiovascular diseases. Men like Balaguer Vintro (Barcelona) and Professor R. Carmena (Murcia) are busy collecting dietary information. Due to the differences of dietary habits between various parts of Spain, it is expected that these studies will contribute to the knowledge of the relationship between diet and cardiovascular disease. One of the difficulties of this type of work is the lack of properly trained dieticians and the same applies to many of the new hospitals. It seems that the preparation of competent dieticians is badly needed in Spain.

Lack of communication among the groups of people working on nutrition appears to be another factor hindering the development of nutrition research in Spain. It is obvious that something should be done to get closer contact and more co-operation between the limited number of persons interested in human nutrition. With the help of others, including myself, Professor Varela is now taking the first steps toward the organization of a Nutrition Society in Spain. I hope this will be a useful step to take.

Whether we will be able to organize a Spanish Nutrition Foundation is questionable. This should be, in my view, the next step if we are to succeed in developing an active Nutrition Society.

Needless to say, I am greatly encouraged by your reports about the activities of the various Nutrition Foundations in America and Europe and, in concluding, I should like to thank all of you for the valuable in formation given in your reports.

Organization and Development of Research in Nutrition in France

André Francois

Director of the CNERNA

I. General Organization of Research in France

The organization of research in France is very centralized. The Délégation Générale à la Recherche Scientifique et Technique (DGRST) is charged with directing research in all fields (exact sciences as well as economy, sociology or philosophy). All research supplies are dealt by the DGRST, except some particular "research budgets" such as those of the Army or of space research, or some estimates at the disposal of universities.

The DGRST is a governmental body directly connected with the Prime Minister. This body proposes programmes and budgets to the interministerial Committee for Scientific Research which involves all Ministers concerned with research.

There are two types of financial aid for research: on the one hand, every year the DGRST endows specialized research institutes in the different scientific fields. On the other hand, the DGRST has at its disposal some particular grants which are designed to encourage sectors deemed to have priority. So this body is disposing of supplies for "concerted actions", the topics of which are clearly defined. Laboratories wishing to take part in concerted actions have to file an application to the DGRST. These are examined by some *ad hoc* committees.

Priorities of research are determined within the scope of the French Five-year Plan. Round tables include researchers and also representatives of professional sectors, of food administrators and sometimes consumers take part in working out the Plan.

So, by a very flexible procedure of self-adhesion, the DGRST has the opportunity of directing researchers towards sectors deemed to have priority and for basic as well as for applied research.

The Seventh French Plan has opted for Nutrition as the first topic for research.

II. Researches in Nutrition

We do not propose to give here a general definition of Nutrition. We have as yet one plain definition coming within the limits fixed by the organizers of this Conference. Nutrition in France includes what is granted by the DGRST. That means that we include in Nutrition, as a part, food technology as well as food toxicology.

Indeed, the policy of the DGRST is to encourage joint work between food producers and people able to direct food productions with respect to nutritional aims, and to encourage joint programmes between, for example, agricultural and medical research.

The Research Institutes responsible for researches in the Nutrition field in France are:

1. the Centre National de la Recherche Scientifique (CNRS), which is attached to the Ministry for Universities;
2. the Institut National de la Recherche Agronomique (INRA), which is dependent on the Agriculture Department;
3. the Institut National de la Santé et de la Recherche Médicale (INSERM), which is attached to the Health Department;
4. the Office de la Recherche Scientifique et Technique Outre-Mer (ORSTOM) in charge of overseas research, is dependent on the Department of Co-operation.

Also, there are research professional institutes, which are principally interested in food technology and food science. These are mainly:

the Institut des Corps Gras (ITERG),

the Institut de la Conserve (Institut APPERT).

III. Role of the CNERNA

The CNERNA (Centre National de Coordination des Etudes et Recherches sur la Nutrition et l'Alimentation) was founded in 1946 by Professor E. F. Terroine. It is attached to the Centre National de la Recherche Scientifique (CNRS) and so to the Ministry for Universities. Nevertheless, the CNERNA is interministerial-oriented since it has been created with the agreement of nine departments.

Its main missions are to suggest to the Government:

1. plans for developing and coordinating researches in Nutrition;
2. programmes for teaching Nutrition (at all levels);
3. basis for the food policy in France in connection with nutritive value of foods;

The CNERNA is, moreover, commissioned for the dissemination of information. At the scientific level, it edits the *Annales de la Nutrition et de l'Alimentation.* For information at a practical level, it has to inform government, industry and consumers of problems concerning Nutrition. This task is, of course, more difficult than dispensing scientific information.

The CNERNA closely collaborates with the DGRST. It is the adviser of the DGRST about anything regarding development of research in the fields of Nutrition, Food and Food Science.

It is also in close connection with departments. One of its main tasks is to transfer results of research towards the utilizers of this research.

On the international plane, the CNERNA is the French adhering body to the IUNS. It was organizer, 2 years ago, of the GEN meeting in Paris.

Beside the CNERNA, missions of which are very wide, there are in France some associations which are interested in different aspects of Nutrition, Food and Food Science. This is normal taking into account the very wide scope of action of Nutrition.

In order to join these different groups, a French Federation of Nutrition Societies is being formed on the initiative of the CNERNA. Among the societies notably concerned is the Société de Nutrition et de Diététique de Langue Française. Another is the Fondation Française pour la Nutrition, founded on Jean Tremolieres's initiative. The aim of the

Foundation is to bring the food industry and the researchers together. Approximately twelve companies are members. Professor Debry is chairman of the Scientific Committee.

IV. Scientific Publications—Scientific Life

Results of research are published in French or foreign scientific journals. In France two main journals publish papers on Nutrition. Let us quote, on the one hand, the *Annales de la Nutrition et de l'Alimentation* which is edited by the CNRS, on behalf of the CNERNA. On the other hand, the INRA edits the *Annales de Biologie animale, Biochimie, Biophysique* which, however, is not only a journal of Nutrition.

Les *Cahiers de Nutrition et de Diététique, L'Alimentation et la Vie* and *Médecine et Nutrition* are other French journals which publish general reviews or original work.

At present, we are changing the *Annales de la Nutrition et de l'Alimentation.* There is now an international editorial board. Moreover, we are advancing towards Franco-English bilingualism.

May I say that we would be pleased to publish in the *Annales de la Nutrition* papers of foreign colleagues, in French or in English.

While waiting for the Federation of the French Nutrition Societies to be set up, CNERNA is playing the main part in the scientific animation. It organizes symposiums or meetings where original papers are presented.

In consequence, we have organized conferences or symposiums on

- May 76: The Human Food Behaviour (published now in *Annales de la Nutrition);*
- December 76: Nutrition Education;
- January 77: Vitamins;
- February 77: The Nutrition of Cold-blooded Animals;
- May 77: Protein Metabolism.

Foreign colleagues may be invited. Professor Swan (St Paul, Minnesota) has participated in the meeting on Education; we had invited

Professor Gräsbeck (Helsinki) to the meeting on Vitamins; Professor Munro (MIT, Boston) has come to the meeting on Protein Metabolism.

V. Distribution of Tasks—Orientation of Researches

A. Distribution of Tasks

Each of the large institutes has its own mission:

- The INRA (Institut National de la Recherche Agronomique) is principally developing research in animal Nutrition. It is yet interested in human Nutrition, in particular regarding the influence of methods of production of foods on their nutritional value.

We have to note that the INRA has to develop, at the same time, basic research on the physiology of farm animals and the practical applications in the animal production field.

- The INSERM (Institut National de la Santé et de la Recherche Médicale) is entrusted with developing human Nutrition.
- The CNRS (Centre National de la Recherche Scientifique) is commissioned to expand basic research.
- The ORSTOM (Office de la Recherche Scientifique et Technique Outre-Mer) is concerned with human Nutrition in overseas countries.

(a) The INRA has created several multidisciplinary research centres. Nutrition and Food are treated within other branches (reproduction; pathology; technology; etc.). However, there is a specialization for each animal species:

- in Nouzilly-Tours (Touraine): Ponetry Nutrition;
- in Theix-Clermont-Ferrand (Auvergne): Ruminant Nutrition;
- in Rennes (Bretagne): Calf Nutrition;
- in Jouy-en-Josas (near Paris) and in Rennes: Pig Nutrition;
- in St Pée (Aquitaine): Fish Nutrition;

- in Dijon (Bourgogne): Human Nutrition and Toxicology;
- in Toulouse and in Jouy: Food Toxicology.

Moreover, a lot of research in technology concerns the "quality" of foods. They are developing in Clermont-Ferrand (meat), Avignon (fruit and vegetable), Nantes (cereals and protein foods), Narbonne (wine).

On the whole, within the INRA about 100 graduates are working in the field of Nutrition and food products.

(b) *The CNRS* has established in Bellevue (near Paris) one research centre on Nutrition, which was first directed by Raymond Jacquot, and now by Alain Rerat.

Additionally, the CNRS is subsidizing some laboratories belonging to universities (Faculty of Sciences or Pharmacy).

On the whole, within the CNRS some fifty graduates are engaged in Nutrition.

(c) *The INSERM.* There is no independent institute of medical nutrition. Research is carried out in research units, for the most part, attached to hospitals. So, Jean Tremolieres was directing, until his death, the Unit of the Hôpital Bichat in Paris. Gérard Debry is directing the Unit INSERM of the Faculty of Medicine in Nancy. There is as yet, within the INSERM, one section of nutrition which is interested in food surveys and in epidemiology of certain diseases (its Director is Dr. Pequignot).

(d) *the ORSTOM* has developed research in human Nutrition for a few years. At present there are two laboratories in Africa. One is located in Senegal; in Dakar, the ORSTOM has been associated with the ORANA (Organization of Researches on Food in Africa). The other laboratory is located in Yaounde, Cameroun. The ORSTOM numbers about twenty graduates in Nutrition.

We have also to note that, in the field of animal research, the Institute of Tropical Veterinary Medicine is working out programmes in different parts of the world.

(e) *Other organizations and the private sector.* Technical institutes have drawn up some research programmes regarding Nutrition (for example, nutritional value of heated oils, ITERG). However, properly speaking these are more concerned with food science than with Nutrition. So it is with the food industry.

B. Main Topics of Research

It is obviously not easy, in so brief a report, to sum up the orientations of research. Nevertheless, I shall try to sum up the most important points.

In animal Nutrition we are most pre-occupied with:

- proteins saving;
- control of proteogenesis and lipogenesis (control of the composition of the animal body).

In human Nutrition the main topics of research are:

- the metabolism of the adipose tissue and obesity;
- the role of food fats in the etiology of cardiovascular diseases.

In food Toxicology, several groups are studying:

- the formation and toxicity of nitrites and nitrosamines;
- the new mycotoxins and the mode of action of mycotoxins;
- the metabolism of chemical additives and drugs.

Overseas, topics are:

- nutritional anaemias;
- estimation of first system of protein deficiency.

This enumeration is obviously too short and does not take all programmes into account.

For the next few years the DGRST has decided to favour the following topics:

1. Human Food Behaviour;
2. Food Toxicology;
3. Relations between Food and the Digestive Tract (in particular digestive cancers);
4. Influence of Technology on the Quality of Foods;
5. Physiopathological Effects of Food (obesity; diabetes; etc.).

I must underline that some joint research sectors are rapidly developing. One example is germ-free life and microbial ecology, and more particularly the function of the digestive flora in animal and in man.

New sources of proteins are also being busily explored, especially textured proteins with the basis of proteins other than soya. A grant of 1.5 million dollars was obtained. We are also developing SCP proteins.

VI. International Relations

There is no systematic structure for international relations. Some French researchers are in close touch with researchers of many countries. In other cases, there is a real organization, as in the field of animal Nutrition, where the European Federation of Animal Production has undertaken to bring researchers closer. For example, symposiums on energy metabolism are regularly organized. The last one was held in France, in Vichy.

Several French nutritionists are members of the Group of European Nutritionists. We also take part in works of the specialized groups of the IUNS.

Different groups of researchers, especially of the ORSTOM, have dealings with the FAO, WHO, or UNICEF. As concerns the EEC, the influence of technology on the quality of foods in the topic of the project COST.

French nutritionists would be happy to be associated in an international effort to improve efficacy of research in Nutrition.

Index